Human Fertility

Henri Leridon

Human Fertility

The Basic Components

Translated by
Judith F. Helzner

The University of
Chicago Press
Chicago and London

Henri Leridon is Maître de recherche,
Institut National d'Etudes Démographiques
in Paris. He is the author of *Natalité,
saisons et conjoncture économique.
Aspects biométriques de la fécondité
humaine* was published by I.N.E.D.-P.U.F.,
Paris.

The University of Chicago Press, Chicago 60637
The University of Chicago Press, Ltd., London
© 1977 by The University of Chicago
All rights reserved. Published 1977
Printed in the United States of America
82 81 80 79 78 77 987654321

**Library of Congress Cataloging in
Publication Data**
Leridon, Henri.
    Human Fertility.
    Revised and expanded translation of the
author's Aspects biométriques de la fécondité
humaine, published in 1973.
    Bibliography: p.
    Includes index.
    1.   Fertility, Human—Mathematical
models.   I.   Title.   QP251.L4213   612.6
77-1913
ISBN 0-226-47297-3

Contents

Acknowledgments

In the first edition of this work, published in French,[1] I expressed my utmost gratitude to Louis Henry, and time has not altered my debt. His name will appear often in the following pages, because more than any other he has contributed widely to the invention and structuring of the concepts involved here.

The present edition, revised and expanded, was made possible mainly by the help and confidence of one person, Etienne Van de Walle, and of one institution, the Population Council.

By inviting me to spend an academic year at the University of Pennsylvania, a most favorable working environment, Etienne Van de Walle gave me the opportunity for many fruitful contacts. Furthermore, he has been an attentive and constructive critic of this work, which is thus also his. By providing financial support for the preparation of this book[2] the Population Council has played a decisive part in carrying out the project.

At a later stage, Robert G. Potter also contributed priceless, meticulous help to the completion of the manuscript.

Judy Helzner, who was in charge of translating the manuscript into English, played a major role, and at the Institut National d'Etudes Demographiques in Paris, Marie-Louise Rolland also played a part by typing successive versions (in French or in English) of some chapters.

I wish to express my deep gratitude to all of these, and I hope they will forgive the imperfections that I was unable to detect or correct.

1. *Aspects biométriques de la fécondité humaine.* 1973. Travaux et Documents, no. 65, Paris: I.N.E.D.–P.U.F.
2. Grant no. D74.70C.

Introduction

Ever since human societies have existed, all human groups have consciously or unconsciously had the objective of assuring the perpetuation of the group and thus of the species. To control the physiological mechanisms for attaining this objective (which were, in fact, poorly understood), man relied primarily on specific social structures and on implicit or explicit norms. For millennia, the individual's freedom of choice was restricted because fertility close to the physiological maximum was required to assure the replacement of each generation. But suddenly, over a period of several decades, or a century at most, the situation has changed.

The "demographic revolution" represents a major step in the field of fertility regulation; however, the distance covered in the knowledge and control of the physiological, psychological, and sociological mechanisms that have allowed, accompanied, or reinforced this evolution in fertility is not as great.

It is true that the physiological processes of reproduction are now well known: from the description of the various phases of the ovarian cycle to knowledge of the systems of genetic coding, science's leap forward has been considerable. Most of these discoveries, however, are quite recent. Let us review some of them.

In the middle of the nineteenth century, several authors "proved" that ovulation took place during menstruation, or just after: (Gendrin, in 1838; Pouchet, in 1842; and Pierre de Bismont, also in 1842). It was only in the first part of the twentieth century that an exact description of the hormonal cycle appeared: the works of Ogino and Knaus on this subject were published between 1924 and 1930.

The next major step was recognition of the role of chromosomes in reproduction, but the exact number of human chromosomes (forty-six) was not made known until 1956, by Tjio and Levan. The first chromosomal anomaly, trisomy 21 (responsible for mongolism), was shown in 1959 by Lejeune, Gautier, and Turpin. During the same period great progress was made in

1

understanding the structure of chromosomes, with the discovery of DNA in 1953 by Watson and Crick.

With the exception of long-known sterilization methods, the use of this scientific knowledge to modify the biological mechanisms of reproduction dates from 1956, when Pincus invented the contraceptive pill. The intrauterine device (IUD) was rediscovered about 1959, though its ancestors had appeared several decades earlier.

However, the major turning point in the evolution of fertility patterns in the developed world is found in the nineteenth century and even, in the case of France, at the end of the eighteenth century. It is therefore clear that individual behavior was modified long before changes could be facilitated by technology: even today, despite great efforts made in the last twenty years, the "ultimate weapon," that is, the perfect contraceptive method (effective, convenient, economical, without side effects) is not known—and perhaps is not even in sight.

But the absence of contraceptive methods in a population is not enough to determine its fertility. Populations may be very different in what we call "natural fertility," as we shall see in chapter 7. Further, the study of these physiological parameters of fertility is a necessary starting point for analyzing the effect of various methods of fertility control. It is to this study that the present work is devoted, using the following approach.

> *Biometry is the science of variability, of the associated phenomena, and of the resulting problems.*[1]

Standard demographic analysis is interested in demographic events as statistical facts, whose interpretation requires various types of information on the individuals contributing to these events (age, duration of marriage, socioprofessional category, etc.). In the case of fertility, the statistical fact is childbirth, which may be simple or multiple, at term or premature, resulting in a live birth or a stillborn child, and so forth. When the event is renewable (as is the case here), the same individual may be found several times, and the analysis grows richer. Nevertheless the principle remains the same; namely, one is interested only in the event itself, not in the conditions for its arrival (or the reasons for its absence). In short, in focusing attention solely on the *impact these events have on the population*, one voluntarily avoids the question of what might have preceded the events among the individuals who make up the population.

My approach here, on the other hand, will be to decompose the process of "fertility" by studying it at the level of the individuals involved. Passing in this

1. E. Schreider, *Biotypologie* 23 (1953): 21.

way from "macrodemography" to "microdemography" is important and useful for two reasons.

First, the influence of various factors on fertility can be understood and evaluated only through the components we will study, because their influence is exerted on only part of these components. For example, we will define a "monthly probability of conception" which is subjected to various physiological or behavioral factors (especially contraceptive practice). This probability is meaningful—and the factors concerned have an effect—only during periods when the woman is susceptible to fertilization, which excludes all periods of temporary or permanent sterility.

Second, if we can then reconstruct fertility from its several components, we are in a position to evaluate precisely the consequences on the macrodemographic level (and thus in terms of standard demographic analysis) of variation in one of the factors—variation which can itself be explained in microdemographic terms.

This way of proceeding, however, is not always worthwhile, for the second step (aggregating the individual data) is not always possible, perhaps because of contradiction in the definition of components or the complexity of the required calculations. Inversely, the fact that aggregation is possible does not prove that the analysis is correct! In particular, the description adopted may not be a unique solution of the problem under study. This may be the case when the analysis is not refined enough: the solution is still legitimate, but only at the level of analysis to which it applies.

Aggregation is possible here, and even fairly simple. Besides the intrinsic interest of this aggregation—for it enriches the analysis of a complex phenomenon—there is an immediate application in a new and important problem. This is the evaluation of the effectiveness of birth control programs in countries where the basic statistics are deficient and, hence, changes in birth rates and age-specific fertility rates cannot be observed year by year. This aspect of the question will not be specifically developed here, but the principle involved will be obvious both from the concept of "contraceptive effectiveness" and from the models proposed.

In general, we must not forget that although fertility is more and more a *social* phenomenon, it is first a complex *physiological* process. Even an apparently simple concept such as the "monthly probability of conception" requires us to refer to specific aspects of this physiology. That is why most of this book is devoted to detailed analysis of the various aspects of this physiology—from the statistical viewpoint of the demographer.

The general structure of the book is the following. The first seven chapters are mostly analytical. After a first chapter which gives a general view of the physiological bases of reproduction, the second chapter presents the framework now classically used by the demographer. Chapters 3 to 6 are devoted to the study of fecundability, intrauterine mortality, the physiological non-susceptible period, and sterility.

This first part is mainly a summary and evaluation of our knowledge, with respect to both the (rare) statistical data that are available on the physiological variables and the demographic treatment of these data. This review has a special interest in itself owing to the wide variety of publications on which it is based. I have had to use a great many journals from different fields as sources: demography, medicine, genetics, biometry, and so forth, and there are no books covering substantial parts of the topic. It seemed useful, therefore, to include a classified bibliography of selected references. This bibliography is by no means exhaustive: in particular, many isolated articles in journals generally unfamiliar to demographers were certainly missed.

The other four chapters represent a synthesis in some respects. Chapter 7 brings together data on the levels of natural fertility, compares them with the results of a model, and discusses the concept of "natural fertility." Chapter 8 generalizes the preceding framework to situations of controlled fertility by introducing contraception, abortion, and sterilization and by discussing the concept of contraceptive effectiveness. Chapter 9 shows how the preceding approaches can be completed by the use of various models, and some examples and results of such models are presented, and chapter 10 provides an overview. A specific example (the study of birth intervals grouped by birth order and final family size) is developed in more detail in Appendix A.

The interest—and success—of the micro-macrodemography distinction is the possibility of moving back and forth from one to the other in a fruitful dialectic: parameters defined at the "micro" level are entered into the model, results (of "macro" level) are compared with available observations, and, in return, this clarifies some aspects of the parameters used. Of course, it is necessary to closely control the hypotheses in order to avoid a vicious circle; but, inversely, the model that required complete and perfect data would be useless—since it could teach us nothing new!

1

The Physiological Basis

A Look at the Physiology of Reproduction

In the human species, fertilization consists of the union of a female gamete (the ovum) and a male gamete (the sperm).[1] The result is the initial cell, a fertilized egg. Fertilization normally occurs in the upper third of the fallopian tube a very short time after the ovum is discharged from the ovarian follicle.

The stock of these follicles, which are already definitely acquired before birth, is large: more than 5 million at the 30th week of embryonic development. However, no more than 450 (that is, less than 1 in 10,000) will mature and expel an ovum during the woman's reproductive career. All the rest progressively degenerate, most of them very early, since there are no more than 400,000 left at birth. In contrast, the supply of sperm is renewed at each cycle of spermatogenesis (see next section).

Each follicle contains a "primordial oocyte," which is a diploid cell; that is, it contains the usual number of pairs of chromosomes (23), all of them identical to the mother's. After its early formation, the oocyte slowly grows in volume, without undergoing cellular division. Starting at puberty, each ovarian cycle is marked by the activation of just one follicle and its oocyte. There then begins a phase of rapid transformations which includes the following stages: after doubling its chromosomes,[2] the oocyte undergoes a first meiotic division, halving the number of the chromosomes (without separation of the pairs). This process yields two diploid cells: one, the first polar body, is expelled from the follicle and resorbed in a manner which is not completely understood; the other cell, called the secondary oocyte, begins a second meiotic division in which the pairs of chromosomes divide and give birth to two

---

1. The principal reference used here is the work of J. P. Gautray (1968, ref. 041). We shall pay special attention to the formation and growth of the *female* gamete.
2. Actually, this phase seems to begin at the time of the oocyte's formation; but the division into two cells begins only at the time of activation.

haploid cells. One of these, the second polar body, is expelled and resorbed; the other is the ovum.

The follicle, which at this point has matured and become a Graafian follicle, now ruptures and discharges the ovum: this is what we call ovulation. The ovum advances along the fallopian tube; if it encounters a sperm during its life span, fertilization occurs. The ovum's life span is known to be short—definitely less than 48 hours, and perhaps less than 24 hours. (The life span of the sperm while in the fallopian tube might be approximately 48 hours.) We must keep in mind that the ovum is in the process of meiosis, and is hence very fragile. If fertilization does occur, the meiotic process will result in the reconstruction of a normal diploid cell—that is, a fertilized egg. In this case the follicle (which has remained on the surface of the ovary and been transformed into the corpus luteum) will continue its activity for several weeks and play a major role in regulating the embryo's early development.

The fertilized ovum continues to advance through the tube, then falls into the uterus (on about the 4th day) and fixes itself on the lining of the uterine wall. This implantation, also called nidation, occurs about the 6th day after ovulation. By this time cellular division has already begun (there are 32 to 64 cells on the 4th day, and about 200 on the 6th day), and so has differentiation of the cells—the process by which a human being is progressively formed. Even if the genetic heritage, and with it all the "codes" necessary for cellular differentiation, are properly inscribed on the initial cell, it is still a long way from this unicellular egg to the completed organism with its several billion cells (which will be viable only after 6 months of development). The following are several stages of this development:

13th–14th day: beginning of the placenta's function of delivering the mother's blood to the fetus (embryo's size: 1–2 mm);

3 weeks: the heart begins to beat;

7 weeks: the fetus manufactures its own blood; the liver begins to function; completion of the brain (size: 2 cm);

13 weeks (3 months): beginning of movement; development of external genital organs (size: 10 cm);

26 weeks (6 months): beginning of viability (size: 25 cm; weight: approximately 1 kg);

38 weeks: full term (average weight: 3.2–3.5 kg).

During this slow and complex process, the risk of accidents seems considerable; and the more we understand about the process, the more clearly we see this risk: "All the biological phenomena [which guide the maturing and survival of the gametes, their fusion, and the early development of the egg] require perfect synchronization in order for their course to proceed normally.... One would be tempted because of this complexity, if daily experience did not prove otherwise, to consider the arrival and success of a pregnancy as very problematical" (Hervet and Barrat 1968, p. 245 [ref. 042]).

Fortunately, there are numerous regulatory mechanisms. Yet certain mistakes, those which affect the genetic heritage itself, are impossible to correct. Such errors may occur at any time during meiosis as well as during early cellular division; and we know that these errors are numerous. Most of the time they are so serious that the egg will not survive more than a few days or weeks. In a small number of cases, development continues and a child is born with mild or serious anomalies (approximately 1% of full-term pregnancies). However, not all congenital malformations are of this origin; one must also consider the effects of harmful (though not lethal) genes, or a nonchromosomal injury to the embryo, especially in the crucial growth period between the 3rd and 10th weeks or during labor and delivery.

It is useful, therefore, to distinguish between congenital malformations, observed by definition at birth in a newborn or stillborn child, which have varied etiology and make up at most only 4–5% of births (including chromosomal anomalies), and malformations observed in fetuses aborted before 20 weeks, which often result from a serious chromosomal anomaly, the frequency of which varies inversely with the duration of pregnancy.

We will return to these categories in studying intrauterine mortality. Let me emphasize here that the process of reproduction is by no means a perfect one, unfolding almost without incident from the moment of fertilization; rather, it is a self-regulating system which corrects its serious failures by eliminating them. The rate of such elimination is high: at least 40%, and perhaps as high as 60%. Although fertilization may take place, it is of no avail in certain cases when the fertilized ovum is defective enough to condemn it to prompt destruction.

Physiology of Reproduction: The Masculine Side

Up to now we have considered only the feminine side of the physiology of reproduction. It is obvious that the woman has a special role to play, since the embryo is formed and develops in her uterus. But focusing attention on the woman is also justified for other reasons, which will be briefly mentioned here.

In contrast to oogenesis, which develops, as we have seen, according to a precise sequence, spermatogenesis is a much more continuous process. On one hand, spermatogenesis also follows a cycle, lasting 74 days, during which the stock of spermatozoa is completely renewed. But on the other hand, gametes at various stages of development coexist at any point during the cycle: the man is normally fecund over the entire cycle, unlike the woman. In addition, although a sperm's period of life (or of motility) is at least 1 week in the seminal vesicle, it is much shorter in the fallopian tube: 48 hours or less. Thus it is clearly the ovulatory cycle that dictates the rhythm of fecundity.

Our knowledge of the bounds of the reproductive period in males is much less precise than our information for females (which will be discussed in the next section). As a group of experts from the World Health Organization have written (WHO 1969, ref. 040a). "there is no clear point at which puberty may be said to have been attained"; and, "the climacteric in the male is a vague and indefinite phase characterized by the gradual decline of spermatogenesis, and the loss of potency and sex-drive."

Puberty is a continuous process which takes place at roughly the same age in men and women; thus, the potential reproductive period begins at about the same time in the two sexes. Also, since men generally marry at an older age than women, the fecundity of a couple marrying very young will probably depend more on the wife's fecundity than on the husband's.

At the other end of the reproductive period, it is generally agreed that men remain fecund on the average until a later age than women.

However, more attention should be given to the masculine side of reproduction. It is evident that what a demographer says about births (or about conceptions) must apply in fact to the *couples* who produced these children, even if the conventional language of demography refers only to the fertility or fecundity of women.

The Reproductive Period: Puberty and Menopause

It is difficult to define the bounds of the women's reproductive period. There are, of course, two objective limits—menarche (which I will call puberty) and menopause (the cessation of menstrual periods). These may be considered extreme limits, since the first menstrual cycles may be anovulatory and since permanent sterility often precedes the menopause (which is merely its final manifestation) by several years.

In 1946 Ashley Montagu (1946, ref. 052) made a remarkable review of "adolescent sterility." Many ethnologists had been surprised by the *rare* occurrence of illegitimate births in populations where premarital relations were tolerated and even encouraged; Montagu considered this fact along with data on the interval between marriage and first conception (when marriage took place *after* puberty) or between puberty and first conception (when marriage preceded puberty) and concluded that there is a period of quasi-sterility which could last several years. This result has been confirmed by several studies in historical demography, when it was possible to calculate a rate of legitimate fertility for women under 20 years of age; this rate is often 10 to 20% below the rate for women aged 20 to 24. It has also been shown that the monthly probability of conception is lower for women under 20 years (see chap. 3).

It is not known whether each woman *gradually* reaches her state of full fecundity or whether this state is reached at a certain point in time, but at different ages in different women. It is possible to try to determine this by studying the interval between first and second births in very early marriages where the second conception could also occur during the "subfecund" period. I have attempted such an analysis with a compilation of data published in various monographs, but with only partial success (see Leridon 1967, ref. 029).

The problem is further complicated by the existence of intrauterine mortality. I have hypothesized above the existence of a phase during which certain mechanisms of the ovulatory cycle (especially hormonal regulation) could be defective; and the consequence of this, as I have already mentioned, is as likely to be an early end to the embryo's development as a failure at fertilization. But whatever the reasons, the phenomenon Montagu described is certainly real.

The age at puberty is often mentioned in biometric studies. Two points to note are: (1) there are great regional and social disparities; and (2) in modern societies, there has been a rapid decline in mean age at menarche during the last hundred years.

For example, let us consider the results obtained by Bourlière et al. for two different groups: upper-class Parisian women (1966, ref. 057) and women of a small town in Brittany called Plozévet (1966, ref. 056) (see table 1.1). We find that puberty is earlier for the former (which illustrates point 1 above),

Table 1.1   Mean Age at Puberty for Girls in Various Populations

Age at Time of Survey (in Years)	Paris		Village of Plozévet (Brittany)	United States	Punjab	Dakar (Senegal)
	Mean	(1) Standard Deviation	(2) Mean	(3) Mean	(4) Mean	(5) Mean
80	13.5	1.7	15.7	—		
70	12.7	1.3	14.7	13.7		
60	13.0	1.8	14.5	13.4	14.5	
50	13.1	1.5	14.2	13.1		14.3
40	12.7	1.2	13.7	13.1		
30	12.9	1.2	13.4	12.8		
Total Number of Cases	268		253	3,581	459	1,317

SOURCES: (1) Ref. 057; survey done in 1957–62.
(2) Ref. 056; survey done in 1963.
(3) Ref. 060; retrospective survey done in 1960–62. A cross-section survey was done at the same time, among 6,710 girls, leading to a mean age of 12.77.
(4) Ref. 063; retrospective survey done in 1955–59.
(5) Ref. 328b; survey done in 1972.

but also that age at puberty for the latter group has rapidly declined: from 15 years, 9 months about 1900 to 13 years, 5 months about 1946. The difference is now about 6 months, where just two generations before it was greater than 2 years. In both groups instances of puberty either before the age of 10 or after the age of 18 are very rare.

Many other authors have mentioned similar results. Table 1.1 also shows the results of a national survey taken in the United States: mean age at puberty was equal to 12.8 years (for 1960–65) and seems to have declined by about 2 years in one century. Tanner (1973, ref. 054) points out an even more rapid decline for various European countries: about 3 years in 100 years, or 9 months per generation. In some countries the rate of decline now seems to be slackening.

One explanation frequently offered for this earlier age at puberty is improvement in nutrition. Frisch and Revelle (1971, ref. 050 and 1975, ref. 040) suggest that puberty is possible only when the individual's weight/height ratio reaches some threshold: the faster the growth in weight, the sooner puberty occurs. This explanation is consistent with the observation that the mean age at puberty seems to be more dependent on social class and economic status than on race (Weir et al. 1971, ref. 055) and that temporary amenorrhea can occur in the case of poor nutrition (see chap. 5).

In conclusion, mean age at puberty is approximately 13 years in most developed countries and probably above 14 years in most other countries. But it is likely that most women are not yet fecund at that age, and that they reach the "normal" level of fecundity only several years later.

It is even more difficult to be precise when dealing with the other extreme of the fertile period. I shall return later to the distribution of age at onset of permanent sterility, trying to estimate it using the proportions of women having no more children after a specific age (cf. chap. 6). This is clearly a "younger" distribution than distributions based on menopause, which I shall discuss here.

Mean age at menopause seems to be more stable than age at puberty, although some authors think it is slowly rising. In modern populations the average age for cessation of menses seems to be 48–50 years (see table 1.2). However, a survey conducted in the United States (MacMahon and Worcester 1966, ref. 060) has shown that about 25% of the women reached menopause early as a result of an operation (such as a hysterectomy); this would tend to counter the tendency toward later menopause mentioned above. It is difficult to make comparisons among different populations since the exact knowledge of age may vary. However, we may still note in table 1.2 the observations on India (columns 7 and 8): to the extent that the ages were correctly estimated, menopause seems to occur approximately 5 years earlier than in more developed regions.

In summary, the total length of reproductive life could be longer than 35

Table 1.2   Distribution of Age at Menopause for Various Populations

Age in Years	United States (1)	United States (2)	Paris (3)	Paris (4)	Paris (5)	Plozévet (6)	Punjab (7)	Villages of India (8)
< 35	0	6	—	—			5	2
35–39	2	7	2	—			15	16
40–44	12	16	28	20			42	36
45–49	44	34	41	39			29	29
50–54	34	32	27	36			9	17
55–59	8	5	2	5			—	—
60–65	—	—	—	—			—	—
Mean age	48.1		~48		49.8	49.0	42.6	
Median age	49.8	49					44	44.8
Number of Cases	897	1,370	228	101	159	124	132	2,976

NOTE: (1) Natural menopause only; cross-section survey, 1960–62 (ref. 060).
(2) All menopauses; cross-section survey, 1960–62 (ref. 060).
(3) Retrospective survey in a public hospice, 1953 (ref. 061).
(4) Retrospective survey in private homes, 1953 (ref. 061).
(5) Cross-section survey among upper class, 1957–62 (ref. 057).
(6) Cross-section survey in rural areas, 1963 (ref. 056).
(7) Retrospective and followup survey, 1955–59 (ref. 063).
(8) Cross-section survey, 1955 (ref. 325).

years if we consider the complete interval between puberty and menopause; actually, however, as we shall see later, the fecund period is on the average only 27–28 years, and in addition both the beginning and end of fertility seem to be progressive processes.

The Ovulatory Cycle

Knowledge of the feminine menstrual cycle is of cardinal importance, since the period during which the ovum may be fertilized is very short (generally given as 48 or 24 hours). The idea of using this characteristic as a basis for contraception was proposed by Ogino and Knaus in 1925–30; however, four types of variation in the ovulatory cycle were soon discovered:
1. the (average) length of a cycle varies from one woman to another (from 10 to 45 days);
2. even for the same woman, the length of successive cycles may vary;
3. the day on which ovulation occurs during any specific cycle may vary;
4. finally, all these parameters seem to change as the woman ages.
In 1956 Vincent reviewed our knowledge of these various sources of variation (Vincent 1956, ref. 049). Today it is acknowledged (see, for example, Matsumoto 1964, ref. 067a) that the "typical" cycle lasts between 26 and 30 days, with a relatively constant postovulatory phase (i.e., from ovulation to

Table 1.3. Distribution of Gestational Interval for Live Births (California 1966, White Births)

Completed Weeks From Ovulation x	Frequency %	Cumulative Frequency from 0 to x (Inclusive) %	Completed Days	Completed Months y	Frequency %	Cumulative Frequency from 0 to y (Inclusive) %
≤25	0.5	0.5	≤181	5	0.5	0.5
26–28	0.4	0.9	182–202	6 (182 to 212 days)	1.0	
29	0.4	1.3	203–209			1.5
30	0.4	1.7	210–216	7 (213 to 242 days)	6.0	
31	0.6	2.3	217–223			
32	1.2	3.5	224–230			
33	1.9	5.4	231–237			7.5

Week	Days	%	Cum. %	Month	%	Cum. %
34	238–244	3.0	8.4			
35	245–251	5.8	14.2	8 (243 to 273 days)	66.0	
36	252–258	12.8	27.0			
37	259–265	21.6	48.6			
38	266–272	23.2	71.8			73.5
39	273–279	14.7	86.5	9 (274 to 303 days)	25.5	
40	280–286	7.1	93.6			
41	287–293	4.1	97.7			
42	294–300	0.5	98.2			99.0
43	301–307	0.8	99.0	10 (304 days and over)	1.0	
44	308–314	0.1	99.1			100.0
≥45	≥315	0.9	100.0			

SOURCE: Adapted from L. M. Hammes and A. E. Treolar, "Gestational interval from vital records," *Amer. J. Pub. Health*, vol. 60, no. 8 (August 1970).
NOTE: Interval counted from the theoretical day of ovulation; i.e., 2 weeks after the first day of the last menstrual period.

first day of the next period) of 14 days (± 2). This could hold for about two women out of three. But even with these regularities, we see that ovulation can occur between the 10th and 18th days of the cycle; hence, the range of uncertainty covers 25% of the cycle.

The frequency of abnormally long cycles is especially high during the postpuberty and premenopausal stages. According to Vollmann (cited frequently by P. Vincent), each of these stages may extend from 5 to 10 years; thus we see one explanation for the subfecundity which characterizes these ages.

Sure to be added to this is the effect of a high proportion of *anovulatory cycles*. However, even outside of these two critical periods, there is a proportion of anovulatory cycles that cannot be ignored. According to Farris (1952) and DeAllende (1956) (as cited by J. P. Gautray), this proportion may be as high as 15%; this can be considered a maximum (owing to a risk of bias in their samples), and other authors estimate the proportion at about 5% (see, for example, J. Pascal (1969, ref. 219) or Collett et al. [1954, ref. 064]).

We may mention here that the curve of a woman's body temperature over the cycle may serve as an indicator. If she has fairly regular cycles, it is possible to determine and then forecast the date of ovulation with reasonable accuracy, according to her *own* statistics. Although this method does not solve every problem, it is a considerable step forward from the Ogino-Knaus approach, which does not take into account information on the day of ovulation.

The Duration of Pregnancy

The duration of pregnancy is, of course, a function of its outcome. The distribution of pregnancies resulting in miscarriages and stillbirths leads to the computation of a life table of intrauterine mortality. I shall return to this topic later and shall restrict the discussion here to live births only.

Table 1.3 shows the distribution published by Hammes and Treolar for California, where the date of the first day of the last menstrual period (LMP) appears on the birth registration form. This table takes into account 198,408 single births occurring in 1966. Here I have subtracted 2 weeks from each interval (so that the length of gestation is counted from the approximate day of ovulation) and have added a section on counting by months (figured at 30.4 days each), which is useful for certain applications.

The mean length of gestation for a live birth is found to be 265 days (38 weeks) when counting from the probable day of ovulation, or 279 days (40 weeks) when counting from the first day of the last period. We may note here that estimating 9 months from "date to date" (for example, from 15 April to 15 January) gives on the average 274 days; depending on the period of the year, the actual figure may vary from 273 to 276 days (cf. P. Vincent 1957, ref. 068, appendix).

The median is very close to 38 weeks (266 days), and the mode is slightly higher: $38\frac{1}{2}$ weeks (still counting from the presumed day of ovulation).

Sex Ratio and Multiple Pregnancies

The sex ratio at birth (number of live boys born per 100 live girls born) is generally about 105 or 106. Although there may be slight fluctuations around these values, any estimates above 110 or below 100 usually reflect either an insufficient number of observations ("random" error) or poor-quality registration of births. It is important, therefore, to control these two sources of error in order to bring to light whatever variations there may be either between populations, over time, with the age of the parents, or in unusual circumstances (such as wars). Error may also result from the fact that the sex ratio for stillbirths not only is subject to wider fluctuations than the sex ratio for live births but is also much higher (currently 120 to 130). Thus, depending on whether stillbirths and live births are correctly recorded as such, the sex ratio may be somewhat higher or lower than usual. (The interested reader may consult section 1.21 of the bibliography for further information on this topic.)

The frequency of multiple pregnancies is relatively less constant. In most countries, approximately 1% of all pregnancies involve more than one embryo, and only a small fraction of these (1%) involve more than two embryos, although the frequency of triplets, quadruplets, and so forth, may be significantly increased when hormones are used in treating sterility or subfecundity. While the frequency of dizygotic twins is variable (cf. James 1972, ref. 263), the frequency of monozygotic twins seems much more stable: about 4 to 5 per 1,000 pregnancies. Fetal death, neonatal mortality, and even infant mortality rates are often considerably higher for multiple deliveries. For example, Cantrelle and Leridon (1971, ref. 023) have observed a mortality rate during the first month which is five times higher for twins than for single births (in a context of high infant mortality).

The proportion of monozygotic twins among all double births may be easily calculated using Weinberg's formula—by subtracting the number of twins of different sexes from the total number of twins of the same sex (since the number of dizygotic twins of different sexes is equal to the number of dizygotic twins of the same sex).

Neither the question whether a pregnancy is single or multiple (which has only marginal relevance for our main topic) nor the sex ratio at birth (which is practically constant) need be given further attention in following chapters.

The Method of Study

This necessary detour into the domain of physiology provides logical support for the choice and definition of the components of fertility. The principles and justification for this method of analysis were clearly developed by L. Henry as early as 1953 (ref. 285) and 1957 (ref. 282).

The existence of the ovulatory cycle, plus the fact that fecundity is not uniform within each cycle, leads to the choice of the cycle itself as the unit of time. Hence, *fecundability* is defined as the probability of conceiving during one cycle, and actually refers not to a woman alone, but to a couple, including the effect of the frequency and distribution of sexual intercourse during the cycle.

One must also clearly take account of intrauterine mortality, that is, the proportion of fertilizations that do not result in a live birth.

Also, as soon as a pregnancy begins, the woman is in a "nonsusceptible" period. The length of this period varies according to the outcome of the pregnancy, and after delivery it is extended by postpartum amenorrhea. Let us define this "nonsusceptible period" as lasting from the moment of fertilization to the first ovulatory cycle or the resumption of intercourse, whichever is later.

Finally, sterility may interrupt or permanently end the fecund period at any time.

Each of these four concepts has an obvious physiological basis. However, it is important to note that each one may also be reached by means of demographic analysis. Both these conditions must be met in order for the method to be efficient.

It is not possible to affirm the full autonomy of these concepts. For example, the border between fecundability and intrauterine mortality is difficult to distinguish; and the end of the physiological nonsusceptible period is difficult to establish because resumption of menses may or may not coincide with the resumption of ovulation. Anovular cycles may, in addition, create at any time periods of sterility that are difficult to integrate into our scheme. I shall return to these points in greater detail.

As for the independence of these four components, there is no reason to assume it a priori. On the contrary, it seems likely that a woman subject to repeated miscarriages would be exposed to a higher risk of premature sterility; or that a high probability of intrauterine mortality would be associated with low fecundability. These various hypotheses have not been discussed a great deal up to now; we shall see, however, in chapter 9, that the problem is worth examining.

2

Components of Fertility in Standard Demographic Analysis

The conventional statistics used in demography mark events that are the product of many components; and it is always difficult to analyze separate components by studying the aggregated product. However, this analysis is not impossible, and the four components of fertility we shall study may be brought to light by means of fairly standard observations.

I shall now turn my attention mainly to "natural fertility," which I shall provisionally define as a situation where there is no birth control through contraception, induced abortion, or sterilization. This concept will be refined and discussed in chapter 7.

From Marriage to the First Birth

In a country where there are few illegitimate births, the beginning of the period of exposure to the risk of conception is marked by marriage. With the exception of premarital conceptions (which we shall investigate later), the date of the beginning of this period can be known exactly. This is a situation found only rarely: it is, for example, difficult to determine after each birth the moment when the woman is once again fecund. The only other means of forming a cohort of women "newly exposed to the risk of conception" is to observe them when they discontinue a contraceptive method which they had been practicing with complete effectiveness. However, even this poses special problems, which I shall take up later.

In the absence of premarital conceptions, the first conceptions would start occurring only during the 1st month of marriage, and the first live births would be concentrated in the 9th and 10th months. The existence of a substantial number of premarital conceptions (they often represent 20–25% of the legitimate first births) is not an insurmountable handicap. Table 2.1 gives the distribution of legitimate first births according to duration of marriage (in months completed) and the monthly rates that result, as observed by Vincent for a group of large families (women married between 15 and 30 years and having had at least 9 live births) (Vincent 1961, ref. 088). We will assume that these women have never practiced contraception.

One may note that the distribution of first births reaches a clear-cut maximum in the tenth period (9 completed months), even though there were a good number of premarital conceptions (at least 25%), and then decreases progressively. Likewise, the series of monthly rates of fertility (the number of births in the month considered, over the number of women who have not yet given birth at the beginning of that month) shows a sharp increase between months 8 and 9, followed by a much slower decline. We will see the reason for this decline later; for the moment, let us consider only the rate for the 10th month.

If all pregnancies lasted exactly 9 months, this rate of fertility would equal the probability of conceiving during the first month of marriage an infant

Table 2.1. Distribution of First Births, per Month, and Monthly Fertility Rates

Completed Months after Marriage x	Number of First Births $(x, x+1)$	Women Still Infertile (at x)	Monthly Fertility Rate q_x (0/00)
0	149	9,920	15
1	248	9,771	25
2	333	9,523	35
3	342	9,190	37
4	407	8,848	46
5	443	8,441	52
6	453	7,998	57
7	319	7,545	42
8	674	7,226	93
9	1,444	6,552	220
10	1,110	5,108	217
11	766	3,998	192
12	586	3,232	181
13	439	2,646	166
14	337	2,207	153
15	255	1,870	136
16	213	1,615	132
17	186	1,402	133
18	144	1,216	118
19	117	1,072	109
20	115	955	120
21	104	840	124
22	93	736	126
23	66	643	103
≥ 24	577	577	

SOURCE: Vincent 1961 (ref. 088), tables XXI and XXVII.

that would be born alive. We shall call this probability "effective fecundability."

In reality, some of the births in the 10th month result from conceptions during the 2d month, just as some conceptions during the 1st month have resulted in births in the 9th month. The compensation is not exact, and the fecundability that is calculated is slightly less than in reality (by about 10–15%), as we shall see in the next chapter. (Compare table 1.3.) I may mention here that an effect of progressive selection owing to the existence of premarital conceptions must also be included. Strictly speaking, the rate at 9 months can be used as an estimate of fecundability only for the women who have not yet conceived during the first 8 months.

From One Birth to the Next

Having thus derived the first component, fecundability, we will now consider a second one: the natural onset of permanent sterility.

It is possible to calculate from a retrospective study of completed families, for each birth order, the proportion of women subsequently fertile (women whose final number of children has exceeded the order considered), called the "parity progression ratio."

The parity progression ratio for order n is calculated in the following manner:

$$a_n = \frac{\text{number of women having had at least } n + 1 \text{ births}}{\text{number of women having had at least } n \text{ births}}$$

The mean final number of children is thus:

$$d = a_0 + a_0a_1 + a_0a_1a_2 + \cdots$$

Table 2.2 Parity Progression Ratios

	England and Wales: Women Married in 1861–70 (Age at Marriage)		United States: Women Born in 1885–89 (Age at Marriage)	
	≤ 20 years	30–34 years	≤ 20 years	30–34 years
a_0	0.965	0.843	0.917	0.612
a_1	0.973	0.911	0.856	0.598
a_2	0.965	0.859	0.754	0.491
a_3	0.957	0.802	0.731	0.460
a_4	0.944	0.726	0.726	0.493
a_5	0.932	0.647	0.714⎫	0.454
a_6	0.915	0.572	0.703⎭	
...	...	...		
a_{19}	0.575			

SOURCE: Henry 1953 (ref. 014).

Table 2.3. Proportion of Women Remaining Childless, by Age at Marriage
(England and Wales, Marriage Cohorts 1861–70)

Age at Marriage	a_0	$(1 - a_0) \times 100$
Under 20 years	0.965	3.5
20–24 years	0.942	5.8
25–29 years	0.901	9.9
30–34 years	0.843	15.7

Table 2.2 lists some values observed in a population still using very little contraception, and in another clearly practicing birth control already.

We note: (1) that the parity progression ratios decrease, but slowly, from one order to the next; and (2) that, on the other hand, the probability of having no children $(1 - a_0)$ and the probabilities of having no more children after a specific number $(1 - a_n)$ increase greatly with age at marriage.

In a population using little or no contraception, the proportion of newly married women remaining childless gives an estimate of the number of women (or of couples) who are already sterile at the time of their marriage, hence at the corresponding age (see table 2.3). It is, in fact, an overestimation, since some women may become sterile after their marriage but before having time to conceive.

Intervals between Births

One always observes (especially under conditions of natural fertility) that the interval between marriage and first birth is shorter, on the average, than successive intervals between births. For example, a typical finding may be: marriage–first birth = 14 months; first–second birth = 24 months; second–third birth = 24 months.

However, each interval contains a mean delay of conception (which varies little, at least early in marriage), and a period of pregnancy (9 months). Hence, we must accept the existence of a supplementary "nonsusceptible period" which follows each delivery and which ends with the first normal ovulatory cycle, when a new delay of conception begins. Thus, the observation of successive birth intervals provides evidence on a third component of fertility.

Conception without Birth

The fourth component is intrauterine mortality. Usual statistics do not permit the evaluation of intrauterine mortality, since civil registration is most often obligatory only for live-born and stillborn infants, and the borderline between spontaneous miscarriage and stillbirth is set, by convention, at 28 weeks of gestation (counted from the last menstrual period), or sometimes at 20 weeks. Thus, it is only by specific data or surveys that the number of deaths before the 28th week can be estimated.

Thus, by various routes, the different aspects of "natural" fertility reach the demographer's attention. And the concepts derived from these observations are uniquely suited for integrating a fifth dimension which has become essential: the control of fertility through contraception (as affecting fecundability), sterilization (as affecting the level of sterility), and abortion (as affecting intrauterine mortality).

In analyzing each of the components separately, we will be looking for the sources of their variations, that is, the factors on which they depend. These factors are of two broad types: *physiological* factors, governing the "natural" side of fertility, and *behavioral* factors, that are within the jurisdiction of the control of fertility.

Yet the distinction is not so simple. Let us take the example of lactation: breast-feeding delays the return of a woman's ovulation through a physiological process. But breast-feeding is also, obviously, a behavior which may be a matter of individual decision or social custom.

The two types of factors thus widely overlap. For the moment, we will keep the above definitions, then return to them when we make the transition from natural fertility to controlled fertility.

3   Fecundability

J'appelle *fécondabilité de la femme* la probabilité que la femme mariée soit fécondée dans le mois, abstraction faite de toute pratique malthusienne ou néo-malthusienne destinée à limiter la procréation.

"I call *fecundability* the probability for a married woman to conceive during a month, in the absence of any Malthusian or neo-Malthusian practice intended to limit procreation."

It was in these terms that Corrado Gini introduced into the vocabulary of demography (Gini 1924, ref. 095) a concept that was popularized only thirty years later by Henry and others. By "Malthusian practice," Gini probably meant complete voluntary abstinence from sexual intercourse; while "neo-Malthusian practice" refers to contraception. We may also mention the fact (taken for granted by Gini) that periods of temporary sterility (i.e., "non-susceptible periods") must be excluded.

Gini gives the unit of time as "a month" without clarifying further; he probably meant a calendar month, not a monthly menstrual cycle. The distinction between the two is often not worth making, since the precision that could be gained would be small compared with the additional complication in the calculations. Such a gain would even be illusory in most cases: as we have noted, the most frequent length for a cycle is 28 days, but the mean length is generally about 30–31 days—the length of a calendar month.

We now need to be a little more precise in our definition because, as we shall see in the next chapter, not all conceptions are recognizable. To be noticed by the woman, a pregnancy must *at least* delay the first menses after conception (modern tests of pregnancy are not efficient before this limit either). Even after these 2 weeks, many women will not be aware of a pregnancy if menses come back within a few weeks. We will thus define:

1. total (or physiological) fecundability, when including *all* conceptions;
2. recognizable fecundability, when excluding pregnancies ending within 2 weeks after conception (first missed menses), following Bongaarts (1975, ref. 093);
3. apparent fecundability, when including all pregnancies recognized and declared (on the occasion of an interview) by the woman;

22

4. effective fecundability, when including only pregnancies ending in a live birth, following Henry (1957, ref. 282).

Figure 3.1 illustrates these definitions. Usually we can measure only "apparent fecundability," and often only "effective fecundability," when pregnancies ended by an abortion of any kind are not known. In this chapter we will consider mainly these two concepts.

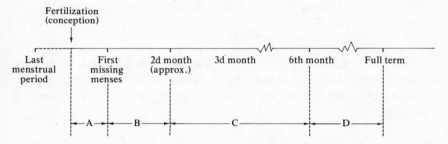

Fig. 3.1. Definitions of fecundability. *Total* (or *physiological*) fecundability: all conceptions; *recognizable* fecundability: pregnancies ending in periods B, C, and D; *apparent* fecundability: pregnancies ending in periods C and D; *effective* fecundability: live births only (period D).

Homogeneous Fecundability: Distribution of First Conceptions

Let us first assume fecundability to be constant and equal for all women in some specific group. Let p stand for this fecundability. We also imagine that all these women marry on the same day; that they have had no premarital conceptions; and that they have no desire to delay their first birth. Ignoring the discontinuous aspect of fertility within the cycle,[1] and assuming that marriage takes place at the *beginning* of the cycle, the first conceptions are distributed, month by month, according to a "geometric" (or Pascalian) law. If N stands for the size of the cohort studied, the number of conceptions will be:

$$C_0 = p\text{N} \qquad \text{during month 0,}$$
$$C_1 = p(1 - p)\text{N} \quad \text{during month 1,}$$
$$C_2 = p(1 - p)^2\text{N} \quad \text{during month 2, etc.}$$

The mean time to conception, m, is equal to:

$$m = 1p + 2p(1 - p) + 3p(1 - p)^2 + \cdots$$

1. Paul Vincent has thoroughly studied the consequences of this discontinuity (Vincent 1961, ref. 088, pp. 168–216), taking into account the fact that marriage could be celebrated more often during the first half of the cycle (before ovulation) or during the second half.

or

$$m = \frac{1}{p}.$$

More precisely, m represents the mean number of ovulations before conception (including the ovulation after which fertilization occurred). The mean time to conception is between m and $m - 1$, depending on the interval that separates marriage from the first ovulation that follows.

The variance of the distribution is also easy to derive:

$$\sigma^2 = \frac{1 - p}{p^2}.$$

Under the hypothesis of homogeneity, the conditional monthly probability of conception, that is, the proportion of women conceiving each month out of those who have not yet conceived at the beginning of the month, is constant:

$$q_0 = \frac{C_0}{N} = p$$

$$q_1 = \frac{C_1}{N - C_0} = p$$

etc....

However, we have seen (cf. table 2.1) that in reality the monthly rates of fertility at durations 9, 10, 11...*decrease* fairly rapidly. This proves that at least one of our initial hypotheses cannot be maintained. The decrease in subsequent rates may result either from a progressive decrease in fecundability during the subsequent months or from a certain heterogeneity among the women with respect to fecundability, the most fecund ones conceiving earlier than the others.

The former assumption cannot be based on a physiological explanation. There is no reason why fecundability would change as an effect of duration of marriage; and the decrease is too rapid to be a result only of the aging of the woman—as we shall see later. It would be easier to grant that the frequency of sexual intercourse is at a maximum during the first months of marriage and tends to decrease thereafter. Existing surveys on sexual behavior (see end of chapter) do not give direct evidence of such a decreasing frequency with duration of marriage, but they do show a decrease as age increases. Here again, the decrease in monthly fertility is too rapid to be accounted for by the variation in intercourse frequency. Moreover, the same phenomenon is seen after each birth, with about the same intensity (see, for example, Cantrelle and Leridon 1971, ref. 023).

Whether this first explanation is true or not—and it cannot be totally rejected—it seems natural to assume that not all couples have the same fecundability, if only for the reason of differences in the frequency of intercourse. Hence I shall consider the consequences of this latter hypothesis.

Before I do so, let us note an interesting point that has been demonstrated by Sheps and Menken (1973, ref. 313, p. 66): If the monthly value of fecundability of any woman is a random variable p, independent from the values of preceding months, the distribution of first conceptions is the same as in the case of a fecundability which is always equal to the mean of p.

The Heterogeneous Case

Gini had already recognized the necessity of taking into account a range of fecundability and had described the process of progressive selection which results: The most fecund women conceive the most quickly, so that the mean fecundability of those who have not yet conceived during the subsequent periods x, $x + 1$, $x + 2$, etc., decreases progressively. Thus the monthly rate of conception,

$$q_x = \frac{C_x}{1 - \sum_0^{x-1} C_i},$$

equal to the mean fecundability of women who have not yet conceived at the beginning of month x, is decreasing when x increases.

The same change may be observed by means of an index proposed by Gini, who was interested in the mean fecundability of women conceiving during a given month (here, month x). This is equal to

$$G_x = 1 - \frac{C_{x+1}}{C_x}.$$

To prove this, we will suppose that the density of probability of fecundabilities is continuous. Let $f(p)$ be this function:

$$\int_0^1 f(p)dp = 1$$

$$\int_0^1 pf(p)dp = \bar{p}$$

Setting the size of the cohort equal to 1, the distribution of conceptions during successive months is the following:

$$C_0 = \int pf(p)dp = \bar{p}$$

$$C_1 = \int (1 - p)pf(p)dp$$

$$\cdots$$

$$C_x = \int (1 - p)^x pf(p)dp$$

The mean fecundability of women conceiving during each of these months is

$$G_0 = \frac{1}{C_0} \int p \cdot p f(p) dp$$

$$G_1 = \frac{1}{C_1} \int p \cdot (1 - p) p f(p) dp$$

$$\ldots$$

$$G_x = \frac{1}{C_x} \int p \cdot (1 - p)^x p f(p) dp,$$

where

$$\frac{C_{x+1}}{C_x} = \frac{1}{C_x} \left[\int p(1 - p)^x f(p) dp - \int p^2 (1 - p)^x f(p) dp \right]$$

$$= \frac{1}{C_x} [C_x - C_x G_x].$$

$$G_x = 1 - \frac{C_{x+1}}{C_x}.$$

The main interest of this formula is that, since it makes use of the *ratio* of the quantities for two successive months, it is not affected much by the competing events that could alter the total number "at risk" in the cohort: death, migration, and sterility.[2] And to avoid having the estimate rest only on a small number of conceptions (those of months x and $x + 1$), Gini proposes using a weighted mean of estimates established for the first n months of marriage: in this way, one obtains the mean fecundability of women conceiving during these first n months and thus belonging to a subsample selected for its higher fecundability. Indeed, Gini proposes calculating the quantity:

$$Q_n = 1 - \frac{1}{\sum\limits_{0}^{n-1} C_x} \left[\sum\limits_{0}^{n-1} C_x \frac{C_{x+1}}{C_x} \right] = 1 - \frac{\sum\limits_{0}^{n-1} C_{x+1}}{\sum\limits_{0}^{n-1} C_x}.$$

Now, the mean fecundability of this group of women is:

$$P_n = \frac{\sum\limits_{0}^{n-1} C_x G_x}{\sum\limits_{0}^{n-1} C_x} = \frac{\sum\limits_{0}^{n-1} C_x - \sum\limits_{0}^{n-1} C_{x+1}}{\sum\limits_{0}^{n-1} C_x} = Q_n.$$

Let us return now to the very first months. We have already seen that

$$C_0 = \bar{p}.$$

2. However, Gini was too optimistic in thinking that his method could be applied without difficulty to contracepting groups. In this case, contraceptive practice may vary appreciably during the first months of marriage and may thus modify considerably the number "at risk" or the level of risk.

The number of conceptions in the first month thus gives an estimate of the mean fecundability for the whole cohort. Also, C_1 gives an estimate of the variance (or dispersion) of this distribution. That is:

$$C_1 = \int p(1-p)f(p)dp = \int pf(p)dp - \int p^2 f(p)dp$$

$$C_1 = \bar{p} - (V - \bar{p}^2);$$

or further, setting $c^2 = V/\bar{p}^2$,

$$\frac{C_1}{C_0} = 1 - \bar{p}(1 + c^2),$$

from which it is possible to deduce the coefficient of variation (c) or the variance (V).

This method, however, attaches too much importance to the events of the first 2 months and leaves out of the estimate a large part of the available information (i.e., the number of conceptions during each of the following months). Later I shall indicate other more effective methods.

Let us end here by stating the values of the mean and the variance of the mean times to conception (with the same definition of this time as previously, that is, the number of ovulations preceding fertilization, including the ovulation during the month when fertilization occurs):

$$m = \sum_{x=1}^{\infty} \int x(1-p)^{x-1} pf(p)dp$$

$$= \int \left[\sum_{x=1}^{\infty} x(1-p)^{x-1} \right] pf(p)dp$$

$$= \int \left[\frac{1}{p^2} \right] pf(p)dp$$

$$\boxed{m = \int_0^1 \frac{1}{p} f(p)dp} \; ;$$

and

$$\sigma^2 = \left[\sum_{x=1}^{\infty} \int x^2(1-p)^{x-1} pf(p)dp \right] - m^2$$

$$= \left[\int \sum x(x-1)(1-p)^{x-1} pf(p)dp \right] + m - m^2$$

$$= \int \left[\frac{2(1-p)}{p^3} \right] pf(p)dp + m - m^2$$

$$\boxed{\sigma^2 = 2 \int \frac{1}{p^2} f(p)dp - m - m^2} \; .$$

If we define a variable λ equal to $1/p$:

$$m = E(\lambda) \qquad\qquad \text{(expected value of } \lambda)$$

$$\sigma^2 = 2\sigma_\lambda^2 + E^2(\lambda) - E(\lambda).$$

Thus, the mean time to conception is equal to the harmonic mean of fecundabilities. It is possible to prove that m and σ^2 are always greater than the mean and variance of the times to conception obtained in the case of a homogeneous fecundability equal to $E(p)$.

Distribution of First Births

In practice, it is usually the distribution of first *births* according to duration of marriage that is used, instead of the distribution of first conceptions. On one hand, we can thus estimate only *effective* fecundability; and on the other hand, the lag between conception and birth alters the calculation somewhat.

I have, in fact, established elsewhere (Leridon 1973, ref. 081, pp. 17–18) that for 100 children conceived during calendar month 0:

2 are born during month 7,
23 are born during month 8,
66 are born during month 9,
9 are born during month 10.

The maximum is reached at month 9, but the distribution is not symmetrical about this month. The result is that the calculation of the estimate is biased for month 9.

To convince ourselves of this we need only return for a moment to the simple case of a *homogeneous* group. Table 3.1 shows a distribution of first births in a cohort of 10,000 women, with the same effective fecundability (0.25) and married at the beginning of month 0. I postulate here that the marriages are uniformly distributed within the menstrual cycle; that is, that the mean time between marriage and first ovulation is about 2 weeks. Moreover, I consider the mean duration of the cycles equal to the mean length of a calendar month. The total of births during month 9 (B_9) is equal to 211 instead of the expected 250. Consequently the ratio $B_{10}/B_9 = 181/211 = 0.857$ is much too high: it should be equal to 0.75, as is the case starting with the following month.

The existence of premarital conceptions would not be sufficient to compensate for the bias, since they are generally too few: 25% spread over 5 or 6 months preceding marriage would make additional cohorts of only 50 conceptions per month in my scheme. Those of month (-1), for example, would yield barely 5 births in month 9, thus raising B_9 from 211 to 216.

Table 3.1. Monthly Distribution of First Births in a Cohort of 10,000 Marriages

Duration of Marriage (in Completed Months) (x)	Month of the Conception and Number of Conceptions									Births B_x	$\dfrac{B_{x+1}}{B_x}$
	0	1	2	3	4	5	6	7	8		
	2,500	1,875	1,406	1,055	791	593	445	334	250		
7	50									50	...
8	575	37								612	...
9	1,650	431	28							2,109	0.857
10	225	1,238	323	21						1,807	0.751
11		169	923	243	16					1,358	0.749
12			127	696	182	12				1,017	0.750
13				95	522	137	9			763	0.748
14					71	391	102	7		571	0.751
15						53	294	77	5	429	

NOTE: Homogeneous fecundability, $p = 0.25$.

We may conclude, from this rapid analysis and from much more detailed investigations of Henry (1964, ref. 098) and Vincent (1961, ref. 088), that the rate of fertility during month 9 underestimates *effective* fecundability by nearly 15% and underestimates *total* fecundability, obviously, by even more.

The situation is not improved during the following months because of the progressive selection in favor of highly fecund women. The rate is generally about the same for month 10 as it is for month 9, then decreases (cf. table 2.1.).

Gini's index (G_x) emphasizes the selection effect even more: the first values are greater than the mean fecundability of the group, and the last ones are smaller. We have, for example: $G_0 = \bar{p}(1 + c^2) > \bar{p}$ (women conceiving during the first month have higher-than-average fecundability).

Beyond the first year of marriage, the distribution of births is not an exact reflection of the distribution of conceptions for an additional reason. If intrauterine mortality occurred only as a "failure at conception" during a given month, with the woman once again becoming fecund the next month, it would be sufficient to multiply the number of births by $(1 + \alpha)$ (with α representing the rate of intrauterine mortality) in order to obtain the number of conceptions. Actually, however, miscarriages occur at various durations of pregnancy, and thus an intrauterine death is accompanied by a nonsusceptible period several months long (3 or 4 on the average) that affects the distribution of live births.

Sheps and Menken (1973, ref. 313, p. 123) have shown that, if μ_w is the mean length of the nonsusceptible period associated with an abortion, α the rate of intrauterine mortality, and λ the inverse of fecundability (with mean

μ_λ and variance σ_λ^2), then the mean and variance of the times to conception for a live-born child are, respectively, equal to

$$m_x = \frac{\mu_\lambda + \alpha\mu_w}{1 - \alpha}$$

$$\sigma_x^2 = \mu_\lambda^2 + \frac{\alpha}{1 - \alpha}(\sigma_w^2 + \mu_w^2) + \frac{2\sigma_\lambda^2}{(1 - \alpha)^2} - \mu_\lambda.$$

The formulas given here apply to the *discrete* case; the variance differs slightly in the case where time is treated as continuous, as was done by Sheps and Menken.

Choice of Distribution Function for Fecundability

The choice of a distribution function depends on the end toward which we are working. We may need a well-defined distribution for specific applications (such as studying the differences between models of homogeneous and heterogeneous fecundability): in this case, we can generally be satisfied with a simple distribution, discrete and limited to a few points, which can be empirically defined. But for estimating the distribution itself from observations, or for constructing a model with continuous functions, we would need to choose a standard function and then estimate its parameters.

Henry has proposed (1961, ref. 079) and then used (1964, ref. 098) a beta distribution (also called Pearson-I). The density $f(p)$ is of the form

$$f(p) = \frac{p^{a-1}(1 - p)^{b-1}}{B(a, b)}, \tag{1}$$

with $0 < p \leq 1$ and $a, b > 0$,

$$B(a, b) = \int_0^1 p^{a-1}(1 - p)^{b-1}dp,$$

which may also be written

$$f(p) = Ap^{a-1}(1 - p)^{b-1},$$

with

$$A = \frac{\Gamma(a + b)}{\Gamma(a)\Gamma(b)}$$

and

$$\Gamma(a) = \int_0^\infty x^{a-1}e^{-x}dx.$$

This second expression is useful in calculations because of a property of the gamma function: $\Gamma(a + 1) = a\Gamma(a)$.

I shall not show the proofs of various results that will be given hereafter. They may be found in some statistics texts as well as in appendixes of articles by Henry (1964, ref. 098), Potter and Parker (1964, ref. 114), and Jain (1969, ref. 100).

First, the mean and variance of fecundability are

$$\begin{cases} \bar{p} = \dfrac{a}{a + b} \\[2mm] V = \dfrac{ab}{(a + b)^2(a + b + 1)}. \end{cases} \qquad (2)$$

It is also easy to define the distribution of first conceptions. The number of conceptions during month j is equal to

$$C(j) = \frac{ab(b + 1)\cdots(b + j - 1)}{(a + b)(a + b + 1)\cdots(a + b + j)}, \quad \text{for } j \geq 1,$$

and

$$C(0) = \frac{a}{a + b} = \bar{p}$$

(the initial size of the cohort having been set equal to 1).

The rate of conception of month j is given by

$$q_j = \frac{a}{a + b + j}.$$

The mean and variance of the times to first conception are as follows

$$\begin{cases} m = \dfrac{a + b - 1}{a - 1} & \text{(if } a > 1\text{)} \\[2mm] \sigma^2 = \dfrac{ab(a + b - 1)}{(a - 1)^2(a - 2)} & \text{(if } a > 2\text{)}. \end{cases} \qquad (3)$$

It is interesting to compare these expressions with the ones obtained earlier for a homogeneous group. Let us assume that the fecundability of the homogeneous group is equal to the mean fecundability $\bar{p}$ of the heterogeneous group. We have seen that, for the homogeneous group,

$$m' = \frac{1}{p}$$

and

$$\sigma'^2 = \frac{1 - \bar{p}}{\bar{p}^2}.$$

By expressing the value of $\bar{p}$ in terms of the parameters a and b,

$$\bar{p} = \frac{a}{a + b}$$

we obtain

$$m' = \frac{a + b}{a} \quad \left(\text{instead of } m = \frac{a + b - 1}{a - 1}\right)$$

and

$$\sigma'^2 = \frac{b(a + b)}{a^2} \quad \left(\text{instead of } \sigma^2 = \frac{ab(a + b - 1)}{(a - 1)^2(a - 2)}\right).$$

In order to extend the comparison, we now need numerical values for the parameters.

Estimation of the parameters

Several methods are available for estimating the parameters. The one in more current use is the method "of moments," which consists of expressing the two parameters sought (a and b) in terms of the first two moments of the distribution (m and σ^2); estimating these moments from the sample; and using these estimates to derive estimated values for the parameters. The formulas are as follows:

$$\hat{a} = \frac{2\sigma^{*2}}{\sigma^{*2} - m^{*2} + m^*} \tag{4}$$

$$\hat{b} = (m^* - 1)(\hat{a} - 1),$$

with m^* and σ^{*2} representing the mean and variance of the times to conception *observed* in the sample. In order to obtain $\hat{p}$ and $\hat{V}$, we need only substitute the $\hat{a}$ and $\hat{b}$ values into formula (2).

In fact, as Majumdar and Sheps have noted (1970, ref. 110), the estimators (4) are slightly biased when the number of observations n is small, since the estimator of the variance σ^{*2} itself is biased. One may avoid this bias by using

$$\widehat{\hat{a}} = \frac{2n\sigma^{*2}}{(n + 1)\sigma^{*2} - (n - 1)m^{*2} + (n - 1)m^*} \tag{5}$$

$$\widehat{\hat{b}} = (m^* - 1)(\widehat{\hat{a}} - 1).$$

In the same article, Majumdar and Sheps proposed estimating a and b by the method of maximum likelihood, then compared the merits of the two methods of estimation. The most important limitation on the use of the method of moments is a practical one: the method requires having available the *complete* distribution of first conceptions (or first births). But in practice these distributions are frequently truncated: for example, the length of observation may be limited to 2 years or may even vary for each woman. In both cases the method of maximum likelihood must be used. Sheps and Menken (1973, ref. 313, p. 98) have given the formulas for these estimators, when data are "censored." Let:

C_y equal the number of conceptions observed during month y (y varying from 1 to t);

N_y equal the number of women who were observed to be exposed to the risk of conceiving during month y;

$$P = \sum_{y=1}^{t} C_y;$$

$$F = \sum_{y=1}^{t} \frac{N_y - C_y}{b + y - 1}.$$

The estimator $\hat{b}$ is calculated by solving

$$1 - \sum_{y=1}^{t} \frac{N_y}{P + (b + y - 1)F} = 0$$

(one may use the Newton-Raphson method for this).

Let $\hat{F}$ be the value of F when $b = \hat{b}$. The estimator $\hat{a}$ is then equal to $\hat{a} = P/\hat{F}$.

These estimators are biased, but to my knowledge the size of this bias has not yet been studied.

Some Findings

The estimates obtained by various authors using the method of moments are shown in table 3.2.

Henry (1964, ref. 098) determined empirically the parameters of a beta function for recognizable fecundability by using fertility rates from the first months as found in a sample of eighteenth-century European populations. Then he returned to a simplified distribution, with approximately the same mean and variance as a beta distribution with parameters of 1.75 and 3.75. Here is that distribution:

Fecundability:	0.05	0.15	0.25	0.35	0.45	0.55	0.65
Frequency:	0.1	0.2	0.2	0.2	0.1	0.1	0.1

$(\bar{p} = 0.320$ and $C^2 = 0.313)$

Potter and Parker (1964, ref. 114) adjusted the data collected in the Princeton survey ("Family Growth in Metropolitan America") for women who

Table 3.2. Estimates of Distributions of Fecundability (Beta Distributions)

Author	Ref.	a	b	$\bar{p}$	$V \times 100$	$c^2 = \dfrac{V}{\bar{p}^2}$	m	σ^2	m'	σ'^2	$\dfrac{m'}{m}$	$\dfrac{\sigma'^2}{\sigma^2}$	$m\bar{p}$
Henry	098	1.75	3.75	0.318	3.33	0.329	6.00	...	3.14	6.74	0.523	...	1.91
Berquo et al.	[a]	2.55	10.65	0.193	1.096	0.294	7.88	252	5.18	21.65	0.657	0.086	1.52
Jain	100	3.48	17.89	0.163	0.609	0.229	8.20	139	6.14	31.57	0.748	0.227	1.34
Potter and Parker	114	2.92	17.34	0.144	0.580	0.280	10.03	288	6.94	41.23	0.692	0.143	1.44
Majumdar and Sheps	110	4.81	14.30	0.252	0.94	0.148	4.75	30.5	3.97	11.80	0.836	0.387	1.20
Vincent	[b]	3.60	11.80	0.234	1.10	0.200	5.54	56.6	4.28	14.02	0.772	0.248	1.29

Meaning of symbols:

a and b are the parameters of the beta-function $f(p)$;

$\bar{p}$, V, and c stand for the mean, variance, and coefficient of variation of fecundability;

m and σ^2 stand for the mean and variance of the distribution of mean times to conception (in months);

m' and σ'^2 would be the mean and variance of this distribution for a group with homogeneous fecundability equal to $\bar{p}$.

[a] Author's calculation, from data published by Berquo et al. 1968, (ref. 092), p. 173.
[b] Author's calculation, from data published by Vincent 1961, (ref. 088), p. 135.

declared no practice of contraception at the beginning of marriage (458 women), and derived an estimate of *apparent* fecundability, as did the next two authors.

Jain (1969, ref. 100) used data collected in Taiwan, with the same qualification (2,190 women married between the ages of 12 and 30 years);

Berquo et al. (1968, ref. 092) collected data in the São Paulo district (2,313 women married between the ages of 15 and 35 years).

Majumdar and Sheps (1970, ref. 110) used data relating to the Hutterites (342 women married before the age of 25 years).

The adjustment of the data relating to the large families studied by Vincent (1961, ref. 088) was made by Leridon (6,552 women having had at least 9 living children).

The last two samples include only live births and thus estimate *effective* fecundability.

The range of the results seems fairly large at first. The *mean fecundability*, for example, varies from 0.14 to 0.32, but it is very probable that Potter's result is biased, since he could not completely exclude the periods of contraceptive practice. Also, the authors did not find it very satisfactory to fit their data to a beta function. Jain also believes his estimate is somewhat low for other reasons; it may actually be less biased than he thinks, however, since the women in his sample married very young (half before the age of 20 years). For the age group 21–25 years, Jain finds $\bar{p} = 0.224$, with a very low rate of registered intrauterine mortality (5%); so this is nearly an estimate of effective fecundability.

From the data of Berquo et al. only the estimates of m and σ^2 have been kept; I have recomputed the other parameters. There are some inconsistencies in the results published by the authors between the values given for m and σ^2 and the theoretical distributions that are supposed to be derived from these values. In table IA, p. 170, the proportion of women conceiving during the first month should be equal to the mean value of fecundability: $\bar{p} = \hat{a}/(\hat{a} + \hat{b})$, $\hat{a}$ and $\hat{b}$ being derived from m and σ^2 according to formulas given above. This is not the case.

The final two groups (Hutterites and large French families) have a mean effective fecundability which is fairly high: 0.25 and 0.23 respectively; but both are representative of populations with unusually high fertility.

The mean time to conception (m) is about 8 months. This is clearly higher than for a homogeneous group, and the difference is greater when mean fecundability is higher. The comparison of variances (σ^2 and σ'^2) is even more striking: in the sample of Berquo et al. the variance is 12 times higher than in the homogeneous reference group ($\sigma'^2/\sigma^2 = 0.086$).

It would also be a mistake to estimate fecundability by the reciprocal of the mean time to conception (as in the homogeneous case). In fact, the product

$m\bar{p}$ varies between 1.2 and 1.9; in order to obtain $\bar{p}$, one must multiply $1/m$ by a coefficient somewhere between these two values of $m\bar{p}$.

It is, moreover, simple to calculate the value of this coefficient in the case of a beta distribution. Starting from

$$\bar{p} = \frac{a}{a + b} \quad \text{and} \quad c^2 = \frac{V}{\bar{p}^2} = \frac{b}{a(a + b + 1)},$$

we find

$$a = \frac{1 - \bar{p} - \bar{p}c^2}{c^2};$$

hence,

$$m = \frac{a + b - 1}{a - 1} = \left(\frac{1}{\bar{p}} - \frac{1}{a}\right)\Big/\left(1 - \frac{1}{a}\right),$$

and, finally,

$$m = \frac{1}{\bar{p}}\left[1 + \frac{c^2(1 - \bar{p})}{1 - \bar{p} - c^2(1 + \bar{p})}\right].$$

It is interesting to note that the coefficient of variation (or its square, c^2) varies only slightly. Bongaarts (1975, ref. 093) has made use of this observation to propose a rapid method of estimating the distribution of fecundability. His model takes into account the distributions of durations of pregnancy for live births as well as intrauterine deaths, yields a rate of intrauterine mortality of 16% during the first years of marriage, and assumes that fecundability is distributed according to a beta function whose coefficient of variation always equals 0.56. Bongaarts proposes estimating mean fecundability by using the ratio of the number of live births occurring between the 9th and 12th months of marriage to the total number of first live births occurring after 9 months of marriage. Several values drawn from his table are presented here as an illustration:

Proportion of first births during fourth trimester of marriage	Mean fecundability
21%	0.10
37%	0.20
48%	0.30

The conclusions that may be drawn from these results, and from various studies of historical demography (see also section 1.5 of the bibliography) are that at about 25 years of age *effective* fecundability usually ranges from 0.20 to 0.25, and recognizable fecundability is probably above 0.30.

Fecundability and Age of the Woman

There are two means of observing the evolution of fecundability with the age of the woman:

1. by comparing mean times to conception, when it is possible to take into

account the age; in practice, it is a question of the time from marriage to first conception, which results in comparing groups that are different in age at marriage;

2. by analyzing the lengthening of the last intervals between births.

This second method, however, does not permit us to draw definite conclusions: since we are considering live births (i.e., effective fecundability only), the lengthening of intervals could just as well be due to a rise in intra-uterine mortality. This is exactly what will be shown in Appendix A.

It would also be possible to ask whether fertility might be a function of other variables associated with age, such as duration of marriage or number of children already born. As early as 1957, Henry (ref. 282) concluded that age itself was the predominant variable, since, under conditions of natural fertility, "fertility hardly depends at all on age at marriage, beyond the first years of marriage." Although this conclusion may have to be qualified today, the predominance of the effects of age remains an established fact.

Let us return now to the estimates based on the time from marriage to first conception. They allow us to follow the evolution of fecundability from puberty to approximately 30 years of age.

Calculating a bimonthly probability at a duration of marriage of 10–11 months, Vincent has found a *doubling* of fecundity between 15 and 20 years, with only a slow increase after that (cf. ref. 088, pp. 212–13). Jain obtains a very similar result by estimating a beta distribution for each class of age at marriage (see table 3.3).

Table 3.3. Fecundability by Age of Women (Taiwan)

Age at Marriage (in Years)	Mean Fecundability	Number of Women
≤15	0.090	69
16	0.093	110
17	0.128	211
18	0.121	292
19	0.151	385
20	0.180	374
21–25	0.224	679
≥26	0.180	70
Total	0.163	2,190

SOURCE: Jain 1969, ref. 100.

The data of Berquo et al., when recomputed, give similar results. Fecundability is increasing from age-group 15–19 (0.187) to age-group 25–29 (0.204) and decreasing afterward (0.191 for women over 30 years).

On the whole, then, the observations are compatible with the hypothesis of an increase in fecundability from puberty to the age of 20. However, we repeat, a certain ambiguity remains: the same result would be obtained if each woman reached her maximum level of fecundability within a very brief time, the age of this transition varying from one woman to another. But in practice this ambiguity has no major consequences.

At the other end of the reproductive career, the situation is different: the very evident lengthening in the last birth intervals of each family (cf. chap. 7) clearly shows a *continuous* passage from fecundity to sterility. In this case, the uncertainty lies in the choice of the parameter: Does the explanation consist of a decrease in fecundability (which could be at least partially a result of a reduction in the frequency of sexual intercourse), or an increase in intrauterine mortality, or a greater proportion of anovular cycles? It is possible that all three play some role and thus that none may be dismissed completely.

Differential Fecundability

Apart from the effect of age, are the observed deviations between the mean fecundability of various groups significant? Before asserting this, we must be aware of a certain number of possible biases:

1. *the memory effect*: the greater the duration of marriage at the time when the woman is questioned about her first conception, the more likely she is to omit mentioning a miscarriage that occurred before her first live birth;

2. *the truncation effect*: the shorter the duration of marriage at the time of the interview, the more likely the sample is to be subject to a selection effect; women with high fecundability have a greater chance of conceiving during a fixed period than other women. This effect works in the opposite direction from the preceding one, though of course the compensation may not be exact.

3. *the importance of premarital conceptions:* in theory, these are excluded from the analysis. But a delivery at 8 or 9 months may result either from a postmarital or a premarital conception, and the distinction is difficult to make.

4. *periods of contraception:* these are also theoretically excluded from the analysis; but in a retrospective inquiry it is very difficult to be sure of the accuracy of the answers on this subject.

5. *the rate of early (nondetectable) intrauterine mortality:* I mention this for the record, since we know as little about differentials in intrauterine mortality as we do about fecundability differentials.

Conscious of all these possible biases, Jain—working from the sample described earlier—nevertheless arrives at the conclusion that, for this sample, there is a positive correlation between fecundability and social status (represented by the level of education, the husband's profession, and the geographic or ethnic origin) (1969, ref. 102). Before concluding that there are real *physiological* differences, according to Jain, we would need more information on possible variations in: the period before consummation of a marriage; the frequency of sexual intercourse; and the desire to conceive the first child rapidly. Thus, as we see, the question remains open.

Another question is whether the examples of results given above (in table 3.2) cover the range of all possible situations or whether some populations might have a much lower mean fecundability, for example, on the order of 0.1. To date such estimates have been obtained only by methods that may be considered uncertain. For example, there have been estimates derived from distributions of intervals between births, which depend on many factors; these other factors not only are as important as fecundability but are even more difficult to measure accurately. Very often, in these methods the mean fecundability is supposed to be equal to the reciprocal of the mean time to conception, which leads always to a downward estimate, as we have seen. However, we cannot reject a priori the possibility of mean fecundability in the range of 0.15–0.20.

If real physiological differences do exist between populations, they could result in particular from major differences in *nutrition*. Just as poor nutrition might increase the frequency of anovular cycles, it could also reduce the fecundability of each ovulatory cycle. A good example of low estimate of fecundability in such a context is given by Menken (1975, ref. 110*b*).

Fecundability after Discontinuing Contraception or after a Birth

Natural fecundability is most easily measurable, in a noncontracepting population, immediately after marriage. In a contracepting population, on the other hand, one must take advantage of periods of discontinuation of contraception each time a pregnancy is desired. Theoretically it is simple to construct, from retrospective interviews, cohorts of women who are "newly exposed to the risk" of conceiving; in practice, it is somewhat difficult to define accurately the first month of exposure for each woman.

This procedure was first applied by Tietze, Guttmacher, and Rubin (1950, ref. 124) to a sample of women consulting an obstetric service in Baltimore. The first monthly probability of conceiving after discontinuing contraception was about 0.30.

Potter and Parker later established, in a comparable study (1964, ref. 114), that the first probability was likely to be highly overestimated, since certain women "rationalize" post facto conceptions which had not, in reality, been planned. They also stated that their estimate was clearly higher than the one they obtained for newly married women (who declared that they did not use contraception at the beginning of marriage). On one hand, there is a risk of underestimation for these newly married women, resulting from periods of contraception which were not declared, but on the other hand there is a risk of overestimation for women discontinuing contraception, resulting both from the rationalization already mentioned and from their deliberate efforts to conceive (efforts which are made effective by the knowledge of the fertile period within the cycle). In addition, it is possible that the estimate of Potter and Parker, for newly married women was lowered by the high proportion of women marrying before age 20 in the United States. Finally, 40% of women were found to have conceived during the month following the discontinuation of contraception, as opposed to 28% during the first month of marriage.

The contraception used by these couples consisted of the so-called traditional methods. The situation is very different after the discontinuation of hormonal contraception or after the withdrawal of an IUD Let us first examine this latter case.

The withdrawal of an IUD has the advantage of determining without ambiguity the beginning of the period of exposure to risk and thus of reducing appreciably the biases pointed out by Potter and Parker. Tietze (1968, ref. 121) has been able to calculate monthly rates of conception after withdrawal of an IUD and has obtained the following values: 0.326 the first month, 0.250 the second, 0.207 the third. In total, 88% of the women had conceived within one year. Of course the sample consisted, at least in part, of women who wanted to have a child.

The situation is more complex after the discontinuation of hormonal contraception. Many authors (see Halbert 1971, ref. 097) have pointed out that for a large proportion of women the first cycles after the discontinuation of hormonal contraception were irregular and even anovular. Unfortunately, in most cases it was impossible to calculate with accuracy the proportion of women subject to these irregularities, month by month, since the authors only cite a total number of cases of amenorrhea or of temporary anovulation. It has, however, been recognized later that some women had had these problems *before* they began to take the pill, which might even have been prescribed for therapeutic reasons. Thus, the effect of the pill has certainly been exaggerated.

However, it is likely that the first cycles after suspension of ovulation are at least irregular. This is the case, in fact, at the time of the resumption of menses after a pregnancy. Pascal (1969, ref. 219) has shown that the cycle *preceding* the first menses was anovular in at least 43% of the cases, and the first cycle *after* the first menses was anovular in more than 10% of the cases —as opposed to about 5% after two or three months. Likewise, the *variance* of the duration of the first cycle was three times higher than that of the fifth cycle. It would thus be easy to accept that the situation is the same after a suspension of ovulation by hormonal contraception.

This is why trying to estimate fecundability after a suspension of ovulation is very difficult whether this suspension results from a pregnancy or from taking the pill.

Another Approach

Up to this point I have considered the monthly cycle as an entity. It is possible, though, to break it up in order to take account of the fact that only a few days of the cycle are fertile and that observed fecundability results from a combination of a "calendar" of the cycle with a "calendar" of sexual intercourse.

The principle of the method is simple. Let N be the number of days in the cycle, minus the menstrual period (for example, $N = 25$); let F stand for the number of "fertile" days in the cycle, assumed to be distributed randomly over the whole intermenstrual period.

The probability of conceiving after one single coitus is equal to F/N, and the probability of not conceiving is $(1 - F/N)$. In total, then, the probability of not conceiving during the cycle is equal to $(1 - F/N)^n$, where n is the number of acts of coitus, and fecundability is equal to $P(F, N, n) = 1 - (1 - F/N)^n$.

We may also assume that the frequency of intercourse is never more than once a day. In this case, the n cases may be distributed in $\binom{N}{n}$ ways over the period N, and in $\binom{N-F}{n}$ cases none of the intercourse falls in the fertile period F. In total, the probability that at least one coitus will result in fertilization is equal to $P_1(F, N, n) = 1 - \binom{N-F}{n} \Big/ \binom{N}{n}$.

The difficulties begin when we try to estimate the parameters. N is fairly well known, and the relative error that can be made in estimating it is not considerable. This is not true for n: the little data available come from somewhat limited surveys and show wide variations with place and age. Though the value of n may be uncertain, the value of the last parameter, F, is undetermined: considering a fertile period of about 48 hours, rather than one of about 12 hours, means multiplying by *four* the most sensitive parameter of the formula. Potter has analyzed very well the consequences of these uncertainties in an article that has lost little of its importance (1961, ref. 113). He relied in particular on results obtained previously by Tietze (1960, ref. 122), and by Glass and Grebenik. ("The trend and pattern of fertility in Great Britain." *Papers of the Royal Commission on Population*, vol. 6, part 1. London: H.M.S.O., 1954.) These last seem to have been the first to propose estimating fecundability by means of the above formulas; Tietze, on the contrary, was looking for an estimate of F, by giving fecundability as about 0.2–0.3. These conflicting approaches show that we seem to be at an impasse, from which only *outside* knowledge will help us to extract ourselves. To convince ourselves

Table 3.4. Probability of Conceiving during a Cycle, by Length of Fertile Period and Number of Acts of Coitus (n)

n	Fertile Period (in Days)						
	0.25	0.50	0.75	1.0	1.5	2.0	3.0
1	0.010	0.020	0.030	0.040	0.060	0.080	0.120
2	0.020	0.040	0.059	0.078	0.116	0.154	0.226
3	0.030	0.059	0.087	0.115	0.169	0.221	0.319
4	0.039	0.078	0.115	0.151	0.219	0.284	0.400
5	0.049	0.096	0.141	0.185	0.266	0.341	0.472
6	0.059	0.114	0.167	0.217	0.310	0.394	0.536
7	0.068	0.132	0.192	0.249	0.352	0.442	0.591
8	0.077	0.149	0.216	0.279	0.390	0.487	0.640
9	0.087	0.166	0.240	0.307	0.427	0.528	0.684
10	0.096	0.183	0.263	0.335	0.461	0.566	0.722
11	0.105	0.199	0.285	0.362	0.494	0.600	0.755
12	0.114	0.215	0.306	0.387	0.524	0.632	0.784
13	0.123	0.231	0.327	0.412	0.553	0.662	0.810
14	0.131	0.246	0.347	0.435	0.580	0.689	0.833
15	0.140	0.261	0.367	0.458	0.605	0.714	0.853
20	0.182	0.332	0.456	0.558	0.710	0.811	0.922
25	0.222	0.397	0.533	0.640	0.787	0.876	0.959

of this, we need only look at Table 3.4, which shows an application of the formula: $P = 1 - (F/N)^n$ to the following cases:

$$N = 25$$
$$1 \leq n \leq 25$$
$$F = 0.25; \quad 0.50; \quad 0.75; \quad 1.0; \quad 1.5; \quad 2.0; \quad 3.0.$$

If we take the approach that Tietze did, and if we keep the limits he set on fecundability (with a preference for the upper boundary, i.e., 0.3), we see that the periods F compatible with frequencies n ranging from 6 to 12 are about 0.75 to 1.0 day. This result agrees with current estimates of the duration of the ovum's survival and would lead us to imagine that the spermatozoon's life span is not much longer. Note, however, that I shall suggest in the next chapter possible values for *total* fecundability (including pregnancies ending within 2 weeks) much higher than 0.3, which should require a fertile period equal to 2 or 3 days on the average.

All this remains quite theoretical, however. A new route has been opened by Barrett and Marshall (1969, ref. 091), who have tried to determine the probabilities of conception by day of the cycle, which amounts not only to defining a fertile period F, but also to weighting each day belonging to F.

The study dealt with 241 married couples, already fertile, mostly Catholic, and practicing the temperature method of contraception. The women were asked to carefully record, besides their daily temperature, the days of menstruation and those of sexual intercourse. These records were required during the periods of voluntary contraception as well as during the time when fertilization was desired.

The day of ovulation is marked on the temperature curve each month. The authors chose as the "first postovulatory day" (index $i = 1$) the first day of rise in temperature. The day preceding this ($i = -1$) is considered as "first preovulatory day."

The authors' steps are as follows. Let α_i be the probability of conceiving on day i, if there has been intercourse on that day. If the probabilities α_i are independent, then the total probability for a cycle of length N is p, such that:

$$1 - p = \prod_{i=1}^{N} (1 - \alpha_i)^{x_i},$$

with $x_i = 1$ if there was intercourse on day i, $x_i = 0$ in the opposite case.

Hence,

$$\log (1 - p) = \sum_{i=1}^{N} \gamma_i x_i,$$

with $\gamma_i = \log (1 - \alpha_i)$.

The coefficients γ_i are evaluated by the method of maximum likelihood, that is, by setting the logarithm of the "likelihood" of the sample of observed cycles at a maximum. The result of the estimate is as follows:

$$
\begin{aligned}
- \log (1 - p) = {} & 0.00x_{-9} + 0.01x_{-8} + 0.05x_{-7} \\
& + 0.00x_{-6} + 0.14x_{-5} + 0.22x_{-4} + 0.19x_{-3} \\
& + 0.35x_{-2} + 0.15x_{-1} + 0.07x_1 + 0.00x_2 + 0.00x_3.
\end{aligned}
$$

Since the standard deviations of the estimated coefficients range from 0.00 to 0.09, the only values significantly different from zero are the coefficients of x_{-5} to x_{-1}. Hence: $1 - p = (0.87x_{-5})(0.80x_{-4})(0.83x_{-3})(0.70x_{-2})(0.86x_{-1}) \times (0.93x_1)$.

In other words, the probability of conceiving, if there has been intercourse on day i, is nearly 0 for all $i < -5$ or > 1 and is distributed as follows during the fecund period:

Day		Probability
Preovulatory	-5	0.13
Preovulatory	-4	0.20
Preovulatory	-3	0.17
Preovulatory	-2	0.30
Preovulatory	-1	0.14
Postovulatory	$+1$	0.07

As we see, each of these probabilities is clearly less than 1. Even after adding one or two times the value of the maximum standard deviation (0.09), none even reaches 0.50.

From the preceding table, we may determine the monthly fecundability resulting from any distribution of sexual intercourse over the cycle. Here are two examples.

1. assuming that the frequency of intercourse is once every y days, fecundability takes the following values, according to the y:

y	1	2	3	4	5	6	7
p	0.68	0.43	0.31	0.24	0.20	0.17	0.14

2. assuming that the frequency of intercourse is z times every 6 days:

z	1	2	3	4	5	6
p	0.17	0.31	0.42	0.53	0.61	0.68

We may note in particular that even if intercourse occurs every day fecundability is not higher than 0.68.

It is also possible to compare these results with the theoretical calculation made in table 3.4 (we need only set $n = 4z$): the agreement is very close, with a duration of the fecund period F slightly higher than one day. In other words, *the set of the daily probabilities obtained by Barrett and Marshall (probabilities of a recognizable conception) would be equivalent to a probability equal to 1 for a little over one day* (and zero the other days).

These results have been established under the assumption that every distribution of sexual intercourse over the cycle was regular. I have also looked at the results under conditions of less regular distributions, for example, assuming two *consecutive* acts of coitus every four days or every six days. For a given cycle, there may be large deviations according to when the group of two acts takes place, within the fecund period, but *on the average* the deviations are insignificant with the model "one coitus every two days" and the model "one coitus every three days."

I have also combined the last table above with a distribution of the frequency of sexual intercourse as observed in a survey made in urban areas of the United States in 1960. (C. F. Westoff, et al., *The Third Child* (Princeton: Princeton University Press, 1963). Here is the distribution:

Frequency per week	<1	1	1 to 2	2	2 to 3	3	3 to 4	4	>4
Number of couples (%)	5.3	15.5	15.7	28.1	8.5	12.9	6.6	4.1	2.9

(Mean frequency: 2.13)

The result is a mean fecundability slightly lower than 0.30. Taking into account an intrauterine mortality of 25%, effective fecundability would be about 0.23; this value agrees well with the available observations.

In the sample of Barrett and Marshall, the method of observation should have been able to bring to light most of the early intrauterine deaths; in other words, the number of conceptions probably is hardly biased at all by the existence of intrauterine mortality (apart from that of the first 2 weeks, which is nearly undetectable), and thus we can regard their estimates as values of *recognizable fecundability*.

As for the effectiveness of the temperature method, we may say that the value of the coefficients $(1 - \alpha_i)$ during the 5 days preceding ovulation, added to the impossibility of predicting ovulation with accuracy, explains the method's high failure rate for any intercourse in the first half of the cycle. After ovulation, on the other hand, the risk seems very low after the third day. But the risk of fertilization of an overmatured ovum, and with it perhaps the frequency of chromosomal aberrations, increases in the days following ovulation.

I have, however, some reservations to the study discussed here. First of all, it is difficult to grant that the moment of ovulation is always determined without error: it is possible that part of the range of the fecund period (6 days) may be due to imprecise knowledge of the date of ovulation. The "true" fecund period could be shorter, with higher daily probabilities.

Also, even though we may consider, as do the authors, that *each* of the coefficients for the values of i besides $-5 \leq i \leq 1$ is not significantly different from zero, this may not be true for their *sum*; in other words, the product of the $(1 - \alpha_i)$ could be significantly different from 1. This is a point which merits examination, before we decide to completely neglect the 20 or so other days in the cycle. Finally, the hypothesis of independence of the α_i could be questioned.

On the whole, this study leaves us with an impression contrary to that of theoretical schemas, in which it was stated that fertilization was possible only during a very short period of the cycle (about one day), and that it took place whenever sexual intercourse occurred during that favorable period. The study described above, on the other hand, seems to show that the fecund period is relatively long (6 days), but that there is a low probability of conception for each day. The growing opinion that fertilization is a process subject to many disorders leads one to believe that this second interpretation is closer to reality, but at the same time we must confess our inability to take into account fetal wastage during the first two weeks.

Sexual Behavior and Fecundability

The preceding analysis has brought to light the potential importance of a behavorial factor: sexual behavior. As was mentioned in chapter 2, it is nearly impossible to isolate purely biological factors and purely sociological factors. We have here a good example of this.

The "disaggregation" of the concept of fecundability, passing from a unit
of time equal to the ovulatory cycle to a unit equal to a day, theoretically
allows a better separation of behavorial factors from biological ones. It would
be necessary, however, to measure the former. The risk of conceiving during
a given month depends, in fact: (1) on the length of the periods of separation
of husband and wife; (2) on the frequency of their sexual intercourse when
they are living together; (3) on the distribution of this intercourse within the
cycle; and (4) on the nature of this intercourse.

The significance of the first factor has certainly been underestimated until
now. In any case, few attempts have been made to obtain quantitative data on
this subject. Recently Chen et al. (1974, ref. 024) have shown that in a rural
zone of Bangladesh the periods of separation could amount to, on the average,
3 to 6 days per month for the farmers, and could even reach 18 to 20 days per
month for the fishermen at certain periods of the year.

Surveys on the frequency of sexual intercourse are fairly rare, and their
interpretation is often awkward. Even if the people surveyed do respond
honestly, it is hard to tell whether they indicate an optimum—or even, a
maximum—rhythm instead of an average rhythm, except perhaps when the
question concerns the week immediately preceding the survey. Be that as it

Table 3.5. Monthly Frequency of Sexual Intercourse by Age
(for Married Women, Husband Present)

Age of Woman (in Years)	U.S., 1970 (1)	France, 1971 (2)	Punjab, 1956–59 (3)
< 20	11.0	—	8.5
20–24	10.1	10.9	
25–29	9.0		
30–34	8.0		5.2
35–39	6.8	7.8	3.0
40–44	5.9		2.2
45–49	...		1.5
≥ 50	...	3.2	
All	8.2		5.0

NOTE: (1) National Fertility Survey: married women under 45. Westoff
1974 (ref. 126). Frequency during past 4 weeks.
(2) National survey by Simon 1973 (ref. 119). The values were computed
from the original data by assuming a mean frequency of 0.2 for women
whose last intercourse took place more than 1 month and less than 1 year
before the survey, and 0.05 for those whose last intercourse took place
more than 1 year before the survey.
(3) Khanna Study (rural Punjab) (ref. 361). The mean values were derived
from the original frequency distribution, by assuming a mean frequency of
13 per month for women declaring one or more act of coitus per week, 2.5
for those declaring at least one per month but less than one per week, and
0.25 for those declaring at least one per year but less than one per month.

may, table 3.5 presents the results of several surveys. In France and in the United States, married women aged 20 to 29 years have declared that they had intercourse about ten times during the 4 weeks preceding the survey. In Punjab the average frequency seems to be about six to seven times at the same ages.

The mean frequency decreases with age—but not very rapidly before age 35. It would be interesting to be able to analyze these results by duration of marriage, at least for the first years of marriage, to see whether the decrease is more rapid at the beginning of marriage.

Indications on the distribution of intercourse within the cycle are available only for some populations largely practicing birth control, and this is linked directly with the study of contraception (the "rhythm" method). It would be interesting to know the distribution in populations that are not controlling their fertility.

Finally, surveys like those of Kinsey in the United States (1948, ref. 107; 1953, ref. 108) or Simon in France (1973, ref. 119) have shown that sexual activity may be practiced with a variable degree of real exposure to the risk of conception. Did not Moheau write, as early as 1778, "On trompe la nature jusque dans les campagnes"?

Final Comment

The difficulties outlined in the last two sections seem to reinforce more than destroy the first idea of fecundability. Certainly, in the course of time the concept has lost its purely "probabilistic" aspect, and it is now clear that it encompasses a much more complex reality than was believed in the past, even in a situation of "natural" fertility. But it has lost none of its operational virtues—indeed, the opposite is true. And we are still a long way from having exhausted its interest, since we constantly encounter new problems in estimating fecundability, and since we know so little about the *real* range of fecundability, whether we consider different populations or simply the members of some group.

Finally, it is already clear that this first "component" cannot be isolated from the others; the border between subfecundity (low fecundability) and sterility is difficult to draw, and the continuity with intrauterine mortality is even more evident, as we shall see.

4   Intrauterine Mortality

It seems unusual that the incidence of a phenomenon which is commonly known and experienced should be largely underestimated, even by those who ought to be most concerned by the subject; yet this is the case with intrauterine mortality. Of course, there are certain reasons for this.

First of all, it is possible (up to a point) for the event to be unnoticed even by the one person who could be aware of its occurrence: the woman herself.

Second, there has been confusion between spontaneous abortion and induced abortion—confusion which persists to a surprising extent. There has been so much attention given the latter that the former has been almost completely neglected.

Third, estimates of spontaneous abortion can vary widely depending on the method of observation and the sampling frame chosen; this is partly a consequence of the first two reasons.

Finally, there is a "trap" that has long been hidden. Accustomed to regular life tables, statisticians have not been aware of an essential difference between the classic study of mortality and the study of intrauterine mortality: in the first case, rates are calculated by relating the deaths to a population of origin that is completely known (a cohort of newborn infants, for example), whereas in the case of intrauterine mortality the population of origin is not known. Even though few miscarriages are recorded during the first month of gestation, the reason is not that few of them occur; rather, the pregnancy is most often unnoticed in such cases. Thus, when the number of miscarriages recorded is related to a number of pregnancies equal to the sum of these miscarriages and of a certain amount of live births, a large number of undisclosed pregnancies (equal to the number of undisclosed miscarriages) are omitted. This point is of fundamental importance and will be developed further.

Questions of Language

Since confusion in terminology can block understanding of our subject, it is important to set some definitions.

The expression "intrauterine deaths" is self-explanatory; it is applied to deaths at all stages of gestation and thus includes stillbirths.

The term "abortion" must be considered ambiguous unless preceded by the adjective "spontaneous" or "induced."

For our purposes, "miscarriage" will be a synonym for "spontaneous abortion." These two expressions usually apply to pregnancies interrupted before the fetus attains viability, considered to be after 6 months of gestation. Beyond this point we speak of "stillbirths."

The duration of gestation may be counted in either of two ways: starting from the first day of the last menstrual period, called gestational interval or conventional duration; or starting from the day when fertilization is assumed to have taken place (which is very close to the day of ovulation), called exact or true duration. There is a difference of about 2 weeks between the two measures.

Life tables for intrauterine mortality are generally constructed according to the duration of gestation at the time the embryo is expelled. Although "duration of gestation" and "age at death" of the embryo are usually confused, we must remember that this is the result of misuse of language, since the embryo may have died well before being expelled. This is why a distinction may be made between "duration of gestation" and "duration of development" of the fetus, the latter being determined by morphological (or other) examination.

The terms "embryo" and "fetus" are here being used interchangeably. Some authors use the former term only for the period between the 3d and 6th weeks of development. Before the 3d week, the term "egg" or "zygote" is generally used.

In most countries the declaration of intrauterine deaths is not required except for stillbirths, that is, beyond 28 weeks' duration of pregnancy (from the last menstrual period), or sometimes 20 weeks. Earlier mortality can thus be estimated only by special surveys.

Problems of Observation

Although studies of intrauterine mortality have multiplied during the last several years, it is, unfortunately, difficult to compare them owing to differences in the manner of collecting data. These differences result in variations that are sometimes large, not only in the estimates of the rate of intrauterine mortality, but also in estimates of the effects of mother's or father's age, pregnancy rank, and outcomes of previous pregnancies.

In fact, we can find at least six different ways of forming a sample of pregnancies in order to study their outcome as a function of several variables.

1. *"Follow-up" survey.* This is the case when we try to discover and follow all the (clinically detectable) pregnancies occurring to a group of women within

a given period of time. The Kauai survey was of this type (Yerushalmy et al. 1956, ref. 162; French and Bierman 1962, ref. 133), as was the Khanna study in Punjab (Potter et al. 1965, ref. 146).

2. *Cross-section survey of pregnancies.* Here, pregnancies occurring to a group of women are studied post facto; these pregnancies become known at the time of the woman's first visit to a physician (for example, through a medical insurance system). The sample may thus be geographically and socially diversified, but the outcome of each pregnancy may not always be known. The studies by Shapiro et al. (1962 and 1969, refs. 151 and 150) in New York City are good examples of this.

3. *Cross-section survey of deliveries.* Often, pregnancies may be known (statistically) only by their outcome, if this outcome must be declared. This is true for New York City, where all miscarriages are supposed to be officially registered, as well as live births. These data have been analyzed by Erhard in 1963 (ref. 131) and by Abramson in 1973 (ref. 127). Stevenson et al. had previously attempted to gather similar data for the city of Belfast (1958, ref. 154).

4. *Survey of pregnancies declared and followed up in hospitals.* This is a classic method of observation; its major disadvantages are that the reference population is unknown and that the women involved may constitute a selected sample of that population. Pettersson studied the pregnancies followed in 1968 at the hospital in Uppsala, Sweden (ref. 145), and Taylor did the same in the Kaiser Hospital in Oakland, California (1964 and 1970, refs. 157 and 158). The results of a study carried out at the hospital of Créteil (near Paris, France) will be given further on (Leridon 1976, ref. 142).

The sample may also select for the *outcome of the pregnancy in question* (e.g., for live births only). In this case, only retrospective data on previous pregnancies may be used (cf. type 6).

5. *Retrospective pregnancy histories in a sample of women.* Sometimes data on all previous pregnancies are collected from the women interviewed in a general fertility study. All this information may be used, with the disadvantages attached to any retrospective study. Jain (1969, ref. 136) studied a sample of this type in Taiwan, and the results of a study carried out in Martinique will be analyzed later (Leridon, Zucker, and Cazenave 1970, ref. 349).

6. *Retrospective pregnancy histories in a sample of pregnant women.* This often accompanies studies of type 4, since obstetric records usually include information on previous pregnancies. Besides the Kauai and Créteil studies that have already been mentioned, we will consider studies by Warburton and Frazer in Montreal (1964, ref. 160) and by Naylor for the United States (1974, ref. 144a).

Each of these methods has its advantages and its drawbacks. Some of these are discussed in my article mentioned above under type 4. To these effects of the chosen method of observation must be added the effects of the method of analysis selected, as we shall now see.

A list of selected studies, with their main characteristics, is given in table 4.6.

Constructing a Life Table for Intrauterine Mortality

From 1953 to 1956 a longitudinal study of pregnancies was conducted on the island of Kauai (Hawaii). The aim of the survey was to record all pregnancies, as soon as they become known to the women, in order to follow their evolution and to draw conclusions from them for perinatal preventive medicine. (General sanitary conditions on the island of Kauai were comparable to those of the United States as a whole.) The most noteworthy idea of two of the doctors involved in the study, F. E. French and J. E. Bierman, was to classify the pregnancies recorded according to the date of their entry into observation, in order to relate the events studied (births and miscarriages), week by week, to the exact number of pregnancies actually affected during the same week. In contrast to standard life tables, the entries into observation are lagged over time: it is impossible for any woman to know with certainty that she is pregnant as of her first day of pregnancy, and the time of the first visit to a doctor varies widely from one woman to another. In other words, we cannot construct a "cohort" in the demographic sense of the term—that is, "a group of persons who experience a certain event within a specified period of time." However, we may best use the available information by constructing a table by the method of probabilities.

Let us call:

A_t the number of miscarriages (or stillbirths) between the durations of pregnancy t and $t + 1$;

B_t the number of live births between the durations of pregnancy t and $t + 1$;

S_t the exits from observation, by the woman's death or departure, between t and $t + 1$;

E_t the entries into observation (pregnancies recorded) between t and $t + 1$.

The number of pregnancies under observation at time t is

$$G_t = G_{t-1} + E_{t-1} - (A_{t-1} + B_{t-1} + S_{t-1}).$$

The probability of aborting between t and $t + 1$ may be calculated according to the following formula:

$$q_t = \frac{A_t}{G_t - 0.5(B_t + S_t - E_t)}. \tag{1}$$

This formula is based on the following hypotheses:

1. The various events taken into account (entry, exit, live birth, miscarriage) are statistically independent. For example, we would have to grant

that the probability of entering into observation is not related to the probability of having a miscarriage.

2. If each type of event were under study alone, their distribution within each interval $(t, t + 1)$ would be uniform.

3. All the probabilities are small.

Under these conditions, formula (1) gives the probability of occurrence of the event studied (miscarriage) *when this event is the only one considered.* From the series of these rates, one may derive a table similar to a nuptiality table: the event studied in this table—like marriage—is not inevitable (all pregnancies do not end in miscarriage), and the principal competing event (death, in the case of nuptiality, or live birth, in the case of intrauterine mortality) ends the risk of occurrence of the event studied (marriage or miscarriage).

We see an indication, however, of an essential difference: both the events studied here (miscarriage and live birth) are really competitive, that is, mutually exclusive; as soon as either one has taken place, the other is impossible. Now we see that formula (1) has a drawback: for pregnancies that last longer than the normal term, the risk of stillbirth increases rapidly; and since a live birth is treated as a "disturbing event," the last rates of intrauterine mortality have much weight in the table, though the real number of these events is small. There are two methods for avoiding this problem: (*a*) we may exclude the B_t term from the denominator, that is, calculate the probability of death *taking into account the competing event*, the live birth (this is the solution adopted by French and Bierman); or (*b*) we may keep the term B_t in the denominator and stop the table at about the fortieth week.

The second solution is not quite satisfactory, although from a theoretical point of view it can be justified by the fact that it is less affected by the choice of time-unit (month, week, or day), and thus the result is closer to the concept of "instantaneous rate," particularly at the beginning of the table. The disadvantage of the first is that it contradicts the usual principle of a life table, that is, that all disturbing or competing events should be excluded; nonetheless, this is the most realistic solution. If we adopt it we must calculate two rates representing the probability of aborting and the probability of delivering a live-born child:

$$q'_t = \frac{A_t}{G_t - 0.5(S_t - E_t)}$$

$$v'_t = \frac{B_t}{G_t - 0.5(S_t - E_t)}.$$

(2)

Thus, we calculate two series of "events of the table," the abortions (a'_t) and the live births (b'_t), and a series of "survivors" (l'_t) who have escaped these two events: $a'_t = q'_t l'_t$, $b'_t = v'_t l'_t$, and $l'_{t+1} = l'_t - a'_t - b'_t$.

The two methods yield, after all, results which are very close to each other, since the difference between the two formulas

$$q_t = \frac{A_t}{G_t - 0.5(B_t + S_t - E_t)}$$

and

$$q_t' = \frac{A_t}{G_t - 0.5(S_t - E_t)}$$

is zero up to the twentieth week ($N_t = 0$) and very small up to the 32d week. After that the relative difference becomes appreciable, but the rates that are calculated become very small in absolute value (at least until the 42d week or so).

Conditions for Use

It is still necessary to make sure that all the hypotheses listed above hold true. The most sensitive part of the table is the beginning: during the first few weeks the "entries" are sometimes distributed quite unevenly over time. In this case, the correction term $+0.5 E_t$ is not adequate at all. This can be shown by calculating separately tables using *weekly* probabilities and *monthly* probabilities (i.e., for 4 weeks), from the same data: the two monthly probabilities derived for the same month may differ by as much as 100%!

The ideal solution would be to work on a *daily* basis. Under certain conditions it is possible to completely avoid the use of correction factors in the demoninator. In the absence of data by days, we may adopt a scale in weeks or even in periods of 4 weeks; but in this last case it would be wise to calculate by weeks for at least the first month of observation.

Another important condition is that the various events studied be *independent*. However, quite often the women who fear a miscarriage are the ones who enter into observation early, while later entries consist only of pregnancies which progress normally and result in a live birth. Also, early medical treatment might avert some miscarriages.

These two points are essential. In a very detailed study, Abramson (1973, ref. 127) has recently brought up these and other problems posed by life tables of intrauterine mortality and has considered four methods of constructing such life tables.

The first method ("cohort life table") consists of distinguishing various pregnancy cohorts according to their duration at the time of entry into observation and calculating a table for each cohort. Although this method is theoretically perfect, the problem in practice is that the number of early entries into observation is always very small. This is precisely why French and Bierman combined all these tables into one—a "fusion life table" in Abramson's terminology.

The other two methods are of debatable significance. In constructing a "period life table," each cohort is followed during only a limited time after the entry into observation, then the portions of a table obtained in this way are combined. The effect of this method is to maximize the correlation between the pregnancy and the date of entry into observation, which may result in a considerable overestimation of the total risk of intrauterine mortality. Abramson obtains a rate of 75% in this way; he regards it as an upper limit, but, as we will see at the end of this chapter, it is certainly excessive.

Finally, the fourth method hardly merits the name "life table," since it consists of combining cohort tables by working as if all pregnancies were recognized at the same time. This is, in fact, the method Mellin had suggested (1962, ref. 143); he seems to have been the first to use the name "fetal life table," although he used it incorrectly since he was not really computing rates by any of the above-mentioned methods. As a result, he found a rate of intrauterine mortality of less than 7%, starting from the 6th week of gestation (counted from the last menstrual period), which is clearly underestimated.

The Available Tables

As I have said, the first genuine table was constructed by French and Bierman and published in 1962 (ref. 133). The calculations—which are reproduced in table 4.1—are done by 4-week periods, using formula 2 (q' and v'). Let us recall the various steps:

1. From the events recorded within each 4-week period (E_t, A_t, S_t, B_t), we calculate the number of pregnancies still in progress at time t:

$$G_t = G_{t-1} + E_{t-1} - (A_{t-1} + B_{t-1} + S_{t-1}),$$

and the following probabilities:

$$q'_t = \frac{A_t}{G_t - 0.5(S_t - E_t)}$$

$$v'_t = \frac{B_t}{G_t - 0.5(S_t - E_t)}.$$

2. From this double series of probabilities, we construct a double decrement table (abortions and live births): $a'_t = q'_t l'_t$ $b'_t = v'_t l'_t$. The survivors (l'_t) who escaped both risks are: $l'_{t+1} = l'_t - a'_t - b'_t$.

In this way we see that of 1,000 pregnancies in progress at (conventional) length of gestation of four weeks, *237 will not end in a live birth*.

If we had been satisfied with the simple method of relating the number of registered miscarriages ($\Sigma A_t = 273$) to the number of live births plus miscarriages ($\Sigma A_t + \Sigma B_t = 3,050$), we would have obtained an "apparent rate"

Table 4.1. Life Table of Intrauterine Mortality by French and Bierman

Gestational Duration in Weeks[a] t	Source data[b]					$G_t - \dfrac{S_t}{2} - \dfrac{E_t}{2}$	Probabilities[c] per 1,000		IUM Table		
	Entries E_t	Abortions A_t	Withdrawals S_t	Live Births B_t	Pregnancies Still in Progress G_t		Live Birth v'_t	Abortion q'_t	"Survivors" l'_t	Abortions a'_t	Live Births b'_t
4	592	32	—	...	0	296.0	0	108.1	1,000.0	108.1	0
8	941	72	1	...	560	1,030.0	0	69.9	891.9	62.3	0
12	585	77	2	...	1,428	1,719.5	0	44.8	829.6	37.2	0
16	337	28	2	...	1,934	2,101.5	0	13.3	792.4	10.6	0
20	248	20	9	1	2,241	2,360.5	0.4	8.5	781.8	6.6	0.3
24	175	8	6	4	2,459	2,543.5	1.6	3.1	774.9	2.5	1.2
28	98	8	4	25	2,616	2,663.0	9.4	3.0	771.2	2.3	7.2
32	67	8	6	72	2,677	2,707.5	26.6	2.9	761.7	2.2	20.3
36	40	9	3	1,074	2,658	2,676.5	401.3	3.4	739.2	2.5	296.6
40	...	11	—	1,601	1,612	1,612.0	993.2	6.8	440.1	3.0	437.1
Total	3,083	273	33	2,777						237.3	762.7

SOURCE: French and Bierman 1960 (ref. 133).

a Completed weeks from last menstrual period.

b Recorded events between t and $t + 4$.

c Four-week probabilities—see formulas in text.

of intrauterine mortality of about 90 per 1,000, or $2\frac{1}{2}$ times less than the "true rate"!

There is a question whether French and Bierman underestimated their first probability (q_4'). The formula used, as I have said, can be misleading if the events are not uniformly distributed over each period. This may well be the case at the beginning of the table (4 to 8 weeks).

To see this, I have calculated a weekly distribution of the "entries" and the deaths, by interpolating on the curves representing the *cumulated* distributions of these events. I have then applied the same formulas as above, but for 1-week periods, and up to the 12th week (as there are no live births yet, the table has only one "exit"; see table 4.2).

Table 4.2. Computation of a Life Table by Week, between 4 and 12 Weeks of Gestation

Week t	$\sum E_t$	E_t	$\sum A_t$	A_t	G_t	$G_t + \dfrac{E_t}{2}$	$\hat{q}_t'$ p. 1,000	$\hat{l}_t'$	$\hat{a}_t'$
4	0	80	0	2	0	40	50.0	1,000	50.0
5	80	120	2	6	78	138	43.5	950.0	41.3
6	200	180	8	10	192	282	35.5	908.7	32.3
7	380	212	18	14	362	468	30.0	876.4	26.3
8	592		32		560			850.1	
4–7		592		32			108.1		149.9
8	592	238	32	16	560	679	23.5	850.1	20.0
9	830	250	48	18	782	907	20.0	830.1	16.6
10	1,080	230	66	19	1,014	1,129	17.0	813.5	13.8
11	1,310	222	85	19	1,225	1,336	14.0	799.7	11.2
12	1.532		104		1,428			788.5	
8–11		940		72			69.9		61.6

NOTE: See text for explanations. One pregnancy was excluded from the 941 recorded between weeks 4 and 11 because the outcome was unknown ("withdrawal").
SOURCE: Data from French and Bierman (1962, ref. 133).

The probabilities for the first 2 months of observation are thus $\hat{q}_4 = 150$ per 1,000 (compared with 108) and $\hat{q}_8 = 72$ per 1,000 (compared with 70).

This calculation is based on a somewhat risky interpolation, but it demonstrates the uncertainty that affects the first probability, which is at the same time the largest. We will return to this result.

In the same year (1962), another important study on intrauterine mortality was published by Shapiro, Jones, and Densen (1962, ref. 151). Although its title mentions a "life table" ("A life table of pregnancy termination and correlates of fetal loss"), this aspect is not much developed, and the methodology adopted for building the table is not clearly explained. The series of weekly rates in its appendix (table VI-A) does seem correct after the 6th week; before this they are clearly underestimated. From the series of these weekly rates, I have constructed a table by 4-week periods in order to compare it with the French and Bierman table. The agreement (see table 4.3) is excellent after about the 8th week, while the rate for 4–7 weeks is quite low: 0.014 versus 0.108.

In 1970, Shapiro, Levine, and Abramowicz (ref. 152) analyzed new data originating from the same source (The Health Insurance Plan of Greater New York) and presented more precise tables calculated by various methods. Two of them have been reported here: a classic table ("fusion life table") and another of the same type in which all pregnancies ending within a week of their entry into observation have been excluded. The size of the difference between the two global rates (340 per 1,000 for the first, 218 per 1,000 for the second) shows the effect of the correlation between the date of entry into observation and the outcome of the pregnancy; but it is difficult to say which of the two rates is closer to reality, since the first can overestimate the true risk and the second can underestimate it.

In 1963, Erhardt (ref. 131) published several tables derived from statistics from New York City. Unfortunately, the formulas used lead to the calculation of *mean rates* and not of probabilities. On the whole, however, the results are fairly close to those of preceding studies.

Taylor has twice used data from the hospital in Oakland (1964 and 1970, ref. 157 and 158) in constructing detailed tables *by week*. This gives us the chance to return to the problem of the distribution of "entries" during the first weeks.

Starting from weekly probabilities (from the 1970 study), it is easy to calculate probabilities by 4-week periods. In this way, we obtain—like the author—$q_{4-7} = 0.0611$ and $q_{8-11} = 0.0487$.

Let us imagine now that the data had been regrouped from the beginning *by month*. By a calculation identical to the one developed in table 4.1, it is possible to determine directly the probabilities by 4-week periods. Table 4.4 shows this calculation.

The first two probabilities are equal to $q_{4-7} = 0.0288$ (compared with 0.0611) and $q_{8-11} = 0.0486$ (compared with 0.0487).

The rate of 4 to 7 weeks is less than half of the result given by the detailed calculation! Thus we see that the question of the distribution of first entries into observation cannot be neglected.

Pettersson (1958, ref. 145) has brought together the results of a series of studies on intrauterine mortality done in Sweden at the hospital of the University of Uppsala. One of the tables he published covers the period 7 to 27 weeks, although not in great detail. Once again, I have recalculated the probabilities by 4-week periods: the probabilities for 8–11 weeks and 12–15 weeks are close to those of French and Bierman (cf. table 4.3).

Table 4.3. Life Tables of Intrauterine Mortality from Various Studies

(Probabilities of death by 4-week periods [q_x], and number of deaths during the same periods for 1,000 pregnancies in progress at 4 weeks [d_x])[a]

Duration of Gestation from LMP x	French Bierman q_x	d_x	Taylor q_x	d_x	Pettersson q_x	d_x	Shapiro et al. (1962) q_x	d_x	Erhardt[b] q_x	d_x	Shapiro et al. (1970) (1) q_x	d_x	Shapiro et al. (1970) (2) q_x	d_x
0									(0.112)	(112)				
4	0.108	108	0.061	61	(0.016)°	(16)°	0.014	14	0.082	73	0.161	161	0.081	81
8	0.070	62	0.049	46	0.064	63	0.059	58	0.067	55	0.135	114	0.081	74
12	0.045	37	0.025	23	0.044	40	0.040	37	0.028	21	0.053	38	0.040	34
16	0.013	10	0.011	10	0.006	5	0.014	12	0.011	8	0.017	12	0.014	12
20	0.008	6	0.008	7	0.001	1	0.006	6	0.009	7	0.007	4	0.006	5
24	0.003	2	0.003	3	ε	0	0.004	3	0.002	2	0.004	3	0.004	3
28	0.003	2	0.004	3			0.002	2	0.004	3	0.003	2	0.003	2
32	0.003	2	0.003	3			0.003	3	0.002	1	0.003	2	0.003	3
36	0.004	3	0.004	3			0.004	3	0.007	5	0.004	3	0.004	3
40	0.007	5	0.004	4			0.005	2	0.011	8	0.002	1	0.002	1
44	...		0.010				···							
48			0.018											
∑Deaths (4–27)	225		150		125		130		166		312		209	
∑Deaths (4–39)	232		159		125		138		175		339		217	

Number of Recorded Events:

∑Deaths(4–7)	32	9	4	92	(About 20)	(About 1,200)
∑Deaths (4–27)	232	571	116	825	—	(About 1,200)
a = ∑Deaths (4–39)	262	729	—	872	(About 500)	
∑Live births (4–39)	1,176	6,809	—	—	—	
b = ∑Live births (4–47)	2,777	15,096	1,069	5,852	—	(About 10,000)
a/b	9.4%	4.8%	10.8%	6.7%	1.2 to 9.1%	12.1%

SOURCES: French and Bierman 1962 (ref. 133); Taylor 1970 (ref. 158); Pettersson 1968 (ref. 145); Shapiro et al. 1962 (ref. 151); Erhardt 1963 (ref. 131); Shapiro et al. 1970 (ref. 152).

NOTE: (1) All pregnancies.
(2) Excluding pregnancies ending in an abortion the same week as the week of "entry."

[a] Double-decrement life table (live birth or fetal death); only the series of probabilities of fetal deaths, and the corresponding number of abortions, are given here.
[b] Life table adjusted and extrapolated by its author.
[c] Week 7 only.

Table 4.4. Recomputation of Taylor's Table by Four-Week Periods

Weeks	E_t	A_t	S_t	B_t	G_t	$G_t - \dfrac{S_t}{2} + \dfrac{E_t}{2}$	q'_t	l'_t	a'_t
0–3	11	—	—	—	0	0	0	10,000	0
4–7	606	9	2	—	11	313	0.0288	10,000	288
8–11	4,770	145	17	—	606	2,982.5	0.0486	9,712	472
12–15					5,214			9,240	

Abramson (1973, ref. 127) has also analyzed the New York City statistics, by studying the effects of the method selected for constructing the intrauterine mortality life table.

The majority of the tables cited above are also given in table 4.3, where one may find: the series of probabilities by 4-week periods, the number of corresponding abortions per 1,000 pregnancies in progress at the beginning of the 4th week, and some indications of the numbers of miscarriages and live births used in constructing the tables.

The differences especially affect the first period (4–7 weeks): if we leave out this period, the series of probabilities are found to be fairly close (cf. table 4.5) (the only divergent case is the one of the second table by Shapiro et al., but this table becomes similar to the others when the abortions occurring in the week the pregnancy was recorded are excluded). The first probability is the highest in the French and Bierman table, and, mainly because of factors related to the method of observation, we may say finally that this table is "the

Table 4.5. Condensed Characteristics of the Intrauterine Mortality Life Tables Cited in Table 4.3

Author	Number of Fetal Deaths (per 1,000 Pregnancies in Progress at 4 Weeks)	
	4–39 Weeks	8–39 Weeks
French and Bierman	232	124
Taylor 1970	159	98
Petterson 1968	125	109
Shapiro et al. 1962	138	124
Erhadt 1963	175	102
Shapiro et al. 1970	339[a]	178[a]
Shapiro et al. 1970	217[b]	136[b]

SOURCES: See table 4.3.
[a] All pregnancies.
[b] Excluding pregnancies ending in an abortion the same week as the one of "entry."

Table 4.6. Characteristics of Various Studies on Intrauterine Mortality

Reference Number	Place of Study	Author and Date	Type of Survey[a]	Number of Pregnancies	Life Table of IUM	Age[b]	Rank[c]	Age and Rank	Outcome of Previous Pregnancy — Only	Outcome of Previous Pregnancy — and Age	Outcome of Previous Pregnancy — and Age and Rank
162	Kauai	Yerushalmy et al. 1956	Retrospective—Women	15,362		×	×		×		
133	Kauai	French and Bierman (1962)	Follow-up	3,050	×						
154	Belfast	Stevenson et al. (1958)	Cross-section deliveries	9,390	—[d]	×	×	×			
151	New York	Shapiro et al. (1962) I	Cross-section pregnancies	6,844	×	×	×	×		×	×
150,152	New York	Shapiro et al. (1969, 1970) II	Cross-section pregnancies	11,630[f]	×	×	×	×		×	×
131	New York	Erhardt (1963)	Cross-section deliveries	2,546	×	×	×				
160	Montreal	Warburton and Frazer (1964)	Retrospective—Pregnant	6,097		×	×	×		×	×
157	Oakland	Taylor (1964)	Pregnant—Hospital	8,041	×	×	×				
158	Oakland	Taylor (1970)	Pregnant—Hospital	15,919[f]	×	×	×				
146	Punjab	Potter et al. (1965)	Follow-up	1,765	×	×	×				
145	Uppsala	Pettersson (1968) I	Pregnant—Hospital	1,258[e]		×	×		×		
		II	Retrospective—Pregnant	3,782[f]		×	×		×		
136	Taiwan	Jain (1969)	Retrospective—Women	9,976		×	×	×		×	
	Martinique	Leridon (1972)	Retrospective—Women	5,672		×	×	×		×	×
127	New York	Abramson (1973)	Cross-section deliveries	247,603	×	×					
144	U.S. Hosp.	Naylor (1974)	Retrospective—Pregnant	33,254		×	×	—[g]			
142	Créteil	Leridon (1975)	Retrospective—Pregnant	3,943		×	×	×		×	×

[a] See explanation in text.
[b] Age of mother; some studies give also the father's age.
[c] Rank of pregnancy.
[d] Data classified by duration of pregnancy. No life table.
[e] 1,258 pregnancies for the life table; 963 previous pregnancies in the retrospective study.
[f] Data of the previous sample are included in this one.
[g] Regression on age and parity.

best." It is worth noting that in this table there are almost as many deaths before 8 weeks as after (108 and 124). Keeping this proportion constant, we see that the various tables lead to a total rate of intrauterine mortality between 200 and 250 per 1,000 pregnancies in progress at the beginning of the 3d week (exact duration).

Age of Mother, Pregnancy Order, and Outcome of Previous Pregnancy

The preceding studies all contain information on the date of entry into observation for each pregnancy, which is somewhat unusual and permits a better estimate of the true risk of intrauterine mortality. In most cases this information is not available, and so we must be satisfied with a "crude rate" of intrauterine mortality (ratio of the number of intrauterine deaths to the total number of pregnancies recognized). This rate is usually between 10% and 15%, as table 4.7 shows.

The following details will aid in the interpretation of tables 4.7 to 4.12:

1. Shapiro's two samples are not independent (the second includes the first), but both are given here since the results were not presented in the same way in the first and second articles.

2. Pettersson's sample I is his prospective survey (chap. 7); sample II, larger, includes all the women who gave birth at the Uppsala hospital from January 1963 to April 1964 (chap. 9). In both cases the data relate here to *previous* pregnancies.

3. Pettersson's samples (especially the first) and Jain's sample all include a fair number of induced abortions. (The overall rate Pettersson observed for his first sample is by far the highest of any.)

4. In the sample described by Potter (Punjab), the proportion of stillbirths is quite high, which is a result both of the small number of *early* miscarriages recorded and of a high incidence of stillbirths (possibly including a number of children born alive but dying before the birth was recorded). The abnormally high rate of mortality observed in the group "under 20 years" is partly a result of the high rate of stillbirths observed in this group.

5. In my sample from Créteil, I have reported here only the retrospective part of the study.

6. Taylor's first sample is included in its entirety in the second sample; thus, only the results of the second article are given here.

Table 4.7 shows the rates of intrauterine mortality by age as given in various studies (I have often recalculated them to make them comparable, for example, by adding figures on stillbirths to Stevenson's rates which had been calculated without stillbirths).

All ages together, the observed rates are between 120 and 155 per 1,000, with one exception in each direction: 196 per 1,000 in Pettersson's sample I

Table 4.7.   Rate of Intrauterine Mortality by Age of Mother (per 1,000 Pregnancies)

Source	< 20 Years	20–24	25–29	30–34	35–59	≥ 40 Years	All Ages
Stevenson et al.	137	109	116	163	183	275	144
Shapiro et al. I	124	97	115	156	....219....		142
Shapiro et al. II	103	108	134	163	....230....		153
Warburton and Frazer	122	143	137	155	187	255	147
Potter et al.	191	121	105	125	171	240	136
Pettersson I	128	181	219	.........242.......			196
Pettersson II	99	133	177	.........210.......			153
Jain	98	83	122	213	286		120
Leridon (Martinique)	101	97	104	139	139	235	121
Yerushalmy et al.	87	68	81	97	122	207	83
Naylor	100	117	141	148	166	255	126
Leridon (Créteil)	129	141	165	193	....247....		154

SOURCES: See table 4.6.

(for reasons we have seen above), and 83 per 1,000 in Yerushalmy's sample (partly because the sample includes women up to the age of 50, for whom the "memory effect" should be important). The most careful observations, based on semilongitudinal observations (not only retrospective) yield rates of about 150 per 1,000: we may thus consider that intrauterine mortality, among pregnancies that are detectable without special methods, is about 15%.

To have a more precise idea of the dispersion of results by age, I have calculated (table 4.8) each series of rates by age, using an overall rate equal to

Table 4.8.   Rate of Intrauterine Mortality by Age of Mother, for a Mean Rate Set Equal to 150 per 1,000

Source	< 20 Years	20–24	25–29	30–34	35–39	≥ 40 Years	All Ages
Stevenson et al.	143	114	121	170	191	286	150
Shapiro et al. I	131	102	121	165	....231....		150
Shapiro et al. II	101	106	131	160	....225....		150
Warburton and Frazer	124	146	140	158	191	260	150
Potter et al.	211	133	116	138	189	165	150
Pettersson I	98	139	168	.........185.......			150
Pettersson II	97	130	174	.........206.......			150
Jain	122	104	152	266	357	—	150
Leridon (Martinique)	125	120	129	172	172	291	150
Yerushalmy et al.	157	123	146	175	220	374	150
Naylor	119	139	168	176	198	304	150
Leridon (Créteil)	126	137	161	188	....241....		150

SOURCES: See table 4.6.

150 per 1,000: for example, if the crude rate was 142 per 1,000, I multiplied all age-specific rates of the corresponding series by the coefficient 150/142.

Although there is no small dispersion in these results, the general tendency is quite clear: from 20 to 40 years, the rate of intrauterine mortality *doubles*, from about 12% to 23%. The increase is especially rapid above the age of 30 years. It is difficult to tell whether mortality at very young ages (before 20 years) is higher or lower than at 20 to 24 years: in six studies out of twelve the risk is higher before 20 years, and in the other six it is lower. These differences could result at least in part from differences in age structure within the group of "under 20 years."

To summarize these results, I have computed an "average series," based principally on the most reliable studies in order to eliminate the most obvious biases. Here we see the mean rates by age, first for an overall rate equal to 150 per 1,000 and then for an overall rate equal to 237 per 1,000 (according to the table of French and Bierman):

	15–19 years	20–24 years	25–29 years	30–34 years	35–39 years	40–44 years	All
Rates per thousand	118	122	135	160	300	270	150
	186	193	214	253	316	426	237

The study by pregnancy order leads to similar results because of the high correlation between rank and age (cf. table 4.9). Again, I have calculated

Table 4.9. Rate of Intrauterine Mortality by Order of Pregnancy (per 1,000 Pregnancies)

Source	1	2	3	4	5	6	≥7	All Orders
Stevenson et al.	107	101	154	168	197	217	210	144
Shapiro et al. I	97	107	138	..........186..........				142
Shapiro et al. II	113	117	146	..........192..........				153
Warburton and Frazer	129	139	130	152	140	188	190	147
Potter et al.	137	143	99	113	....130.....		170	136
Pettersson I	159	217	316	318	........179......			196
Pettersson II	112	180	235	199	200	205	320	153
Jain[a]	86	109	99	148	189	240	345	165
Leridon (Martinique)	98	103	110	108	127	107	167	121
Yerushalmy et al.	80	82	79	....84...		87[b]	120[c]	83
Leridon (Créteil)	153	172	161	.......130.....			—	154

SOURCES: See table 4.6.
[a] Series *estimated* by Jain.
[b] Orders 6–7.
[c] Orders 8 and over.

Table 4.10.   Rate of Intrauterine Mortality by Order of Pregnancy, for a Mean Rate Set Equal to 150 per 1,000

Source	1	2	3	4	5	6	≥7	All Orders
Stevenson et al.	111	105	160	175	205	226	219	150
Shapiro et al. I	102	113	146	...........196..........				150
Shapiro et al. II	111	115	143	...........188..........				150
Warburton and Frazer	132	142	133	155	143	192	194	150
Potter et al.	151	158	109	125	....143...		187	150
Pettersson I	122	166	242	243	........137.......			150
Pettersson II	110	176	230	195	196	201	314	150
Jain[a]	78	99	90	135	172	218	314	150
Leridon (Martinique)	121	128	136	134	157	133	207	150
Yerushalmy et al.	144	148	143	...152...		157	217	150
Leridon (Créteil)	149	167	157	.......127......			—	150

SOURCES: See table 4.6.
[a] Series *estimated* by Jain.

comparative rates based on an overall mortality of 15%. But this time (table 4.10) the range of results is much larger, and it would be risky to define a series of mean rates. However, we may note that the spread is not very wide *for order 1*: thus it seems that the "starting rate," that is, at the beginning of fertile life, may not vary much from one group to another. What happens afterward that causes the spread to increase? Only longitudinal observation of successive pregnancies could help us to better understand this evolution.

The manner of considering previous reproductive histories varies greatly from one study to another. Table 4.11 shows some available results, by outcome of the pregnancy immediately preceding the pregnancy observed in the study, and by the number of miscarriages among all previous pregnancies. The most striking result is the *doubling* of the risk of miscarriage once the woman has had at least one, and especially immediately after a pregnancy ended by a miscarriage. This is a fundamental finding which will be studied in greater detail further on.

Let us note, finally, that intrauterine mortality *increases with the age of the mother even for first-order pregnancies*, which proves that age plays a role independent of rank and of previous reproductive history (table 4.12). At each age, the rate for pregnancies of rank 1 is generally a bit less than the rate for "all ranks combined," which is consistent with the above conclusion on the increase of risk after a miscarriage. We note that for the group "35 years and over" the rate of mortality for the first rank is systematically higher than the rate at other ranks; on one hand, it is likely that the mean age of primi-parous women within this group is less than the mean age of multiparous

Table 4.11. Rate of Intrauterine Mortality by Outcome of Previous Pregnancies (per 1,000 Pregnancies)

	No Previous Pregnancy	Previous Pregnancy		Number of Fetal Deaths among All Previous Pregnancies				
		Live Birth	Fetal Death	0	1	2	3+	1+
Shapiro I	97	110	222					
Shapiro II	113	129	232	126				219
Warburton	129		267[a]	123	237	262	317	248
Pettersson I	159			225	343	......333......		
Pettersson II	112		244	179	268	415	400	
Leridon (Martinique)	98	104	203[a,b]	88[b]	189[b]	......247[b]......		201[b]
Yerushalmy et al.		70	129[c]	70	114	......153......		
Leridon (Créteil)	155	151	266[b]	152[b]	220[b]	353[b]	—	

SOURCES: See table 4.6.
[a] Rate after the *first* abortion.
[b] Orders 1 to 6 only.
[c] Previous pregnancy was an abortion after 20 weeks.

Table 4.12. Rate of Intrauterine Mortality by Age for First Pregnancy, and for All Pregnancies (per 1,000 Pregnancies)

	Rank	< 20 Years	20–24	25–29	30–34	≥ 35 Years	All Ages
Stevenson	1	127	91	91	152	214	107
	All	137	109	116	163	206	144
Shapiro I	1	126	80	72	130	262	97
	All	124	97	115	156	219	142
Shapiro II	1		....94.....		151	277	113
	All		...124.....		163	230	153
Warburton	1	106	142	102	173	(471)	129
	All	122	143	137	155	199	147
Leridon	1	87	89	121	145	188	98
(Martinique)	All	101	97	104	139	167	121
Leridon	1	134	142	177	.....333....		153
(Créteil)	All	129	141	165	193	247	154

SOURCES: See table 4.6.

women. But, on the other hand, the primiparous women over 35 years of age must be a group which has been selected for by previous difficulty in conceiving. Thus, it is hard to say whether the observed deviation is significant.

Study of Successive Pregnancies

The following analysis is the result of a study carried out in 1968 on Martinique, on a sample representing the female population of the island from ages 15 to 54. The list of successive pregnancies was obtained by simple retrospective interviews, but the consistency of results with nonretrospective studies attests to the quality of these data. Another index of the care with which the interviewers conducted this part of the investigation has already been furnished by the study—a priori even more difficult—of fertility in relation to the type and timing of unions (cf. Leridon 1971, ref. 348). Also I have calculated the rates of intrauterine mortality by rank for each generation (i.e., for each group of age at the time of the survey) to show any biases related to the interval elapsed between the first events (first pregnancies) and the date of observation. No significant deviations were found.

As for the list of pregnancies, the survey benefited from favorable conditions on Martinique: there is a good official registration system for births, and most women participate in the French system of maternity health insurance. All this was still within the framework of a society with little regulation of fertility during the period considered.

Table 4.13. Martinique: Intrauterine Mortality by Rank of Pregnancy and Age of Mother

Rank of Pregnancy	Outcome[a]	Age of Mother						All Ages
		< 20	20–24	25–29	30–34	35–39	40–44	
1	SA	32	39	21	8	2	1	103
	LB+SA	369	437	174	55	14	2	1051
	Rate	0.087	0.089	0.121	......0.155........			0.098
2	SA	17	44	18	6	7	1	93
	LB+SA	140	406	254	82	20	5	907
	Rate	0.121	0.108	0.071	......0.131........			0.103
3 and 4	SA	6	43	52	42	10	4	157
	LB+SA	36	455	560	301	73	14	1439
	Rate		0.095	0.093	0.140	...0.161....		0.109
5 and more	SA	0	11	66	109	82	63	331
	LB+SA	1	110	528	746	618	272	2275
	Rate		0.100	0.125	0.146	0.133	0.232	0.145
All Ranks	SA	55	137	157	165	101	69	684
	LB+SA	546	1408	1516	1184	725	293	5672
	Rate	0.101	0.097	0.104	0.139	0.139	0.235	0.121

[a] SA = spontaneous abortion (or stillbirth); LB = live birth.

I have already given, in tables 4.9 and 4.10, the rates of intrauterine mortality by age or by rank which resulted from this sample. (The sample size used here is 5,672 pregnancies.) Rates by age and rank combined can be found in table 4.13 and figure 4.1. (The mother's age is always counted at the end of the pregnancy.)

I have also calculated rates by age, rank, and outcome of previous pregnancy. Overall, for ranks 2 through 10 the risk of miscarriage after a live birth is 104 per 1,000, while it jumps to *244 per 1,000* after a miscarriage. The ratio between these two risks is a bit smaller at young ages and for ranks 3 and 4, but it always remains over 1.5 (table 4.14). Limiting ourselves to second-order pregnancies occurring before 25 years, we obtain the following rates: after a live birth: 47/498 = 9.4% miscarriage; after a miscarriage: 14/47 = 29.8% miscarriage.

To continue this analysis, I have systematically investigated successive pregnancies for ranks 1 to 6. Only these first six ranks (including 4,406 pregnancies, or 78% of the total) were considered, for the following reasons:

a. For a woman who has had 6 pregnancies, the number of possible "reproductive histories" is equal to 2^6, or 64; beyond the sixth rank, the number of possible combinations rapidly exceeds the number of pregnancies observed for the same rank, and the results are no longer valid. In practice, we should sometimes use only the first four ranks.

b. The age effect is reduced, since the sample of the first six pregnancies

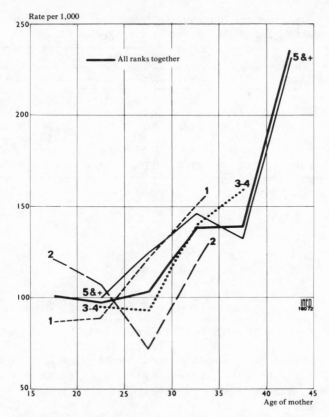

Fig. 4.1. Intrauterine mortality by age of mother and pregnancy order (Martinique).

contains only 31% over 35 years, and that of the first four pregnancies contains only 4%.

The complete "tree" of these 4,406 pregnancies by rank has been constructed and is reproduced here (fig. 4.2). (It was also broken down into three parts by age at the end of each pregnancy: under 25 years, 25 to 34 years, and 35 years and over.) Figure 4.3 summarizes the principal results, which will be further developed here. The overall proportion of miscarriages among the pregnancies of ranks 1 to 6 is found to be 10.7% (472/4,406).

For the first pregnancy, the risk of miscarriage is, as we have seen, 9.8%. If this pregnancy is carried to term normally, the risk remains approximately the same for the following rank (72/824 = 8.7%); and likewise for rank 3, after two live births (64/654 = 9.8%). On the other hand, after a miscarriage at rank 1 the risk increases to 25.3% (21/83) for rank 2 and seems even higher

Table 4.14. Martinique: Intrauterine Mortality by Outcome of Previous Pregnancy and by Age or Rank

Previous Pregnancy	Current Pregnancy[a]	Age of Mother						All Ages
		15–19	20–24	25–29	30–34	35–39	≥40	
LB	SA	19	83	111	101	58	34	406
	SA+LB	156	878	1,211	951	534	167	3897
	Rate	0.122	0.095	0.092	0.106	0.109	0.204	0.104
SA	SA	4	15	23	42	15	9	108
	SA+LB	21	92	125	126	56	22	442
	Rate	0.190	0.163	0.184	0.333	0.268	0.409	0.244

		Rank of Current Pregnancy					All Ranks
		2	3	4	5	6–10	
LB	SA	72	72	60	54	148	406
	SA+LB	823	705	592	501	1,296	3,897
	Rate	0.087	0.102	0.101	0.108	0.116	0.104
SA	SA	21	13	12	17	45	108
	SA+LB	83	67	73	59	160	442
	Rate	0.253	0.194	0.164	0.288	0.281	0.244

[a] SA = spontaneous abortion (or stillbirth); LB = live birth.

after two successive miscarriages at ranks 1 and 2 (5/17 = 29.4% for rank 3, or 19/56 = 33.9% for ranks 3 to 6 combined). In general, the risk of a first miscarriage remains low (under 10%) when live births follow one another (see table 4.15).

The fact that the risk of having a first miscarriage tends to decrease as the pregnancy rank increases leads us to believe that there is a selection process: women with high risk become fewer and fewer from one line of the previous table to the next. The decrease is fairly slow, however, perhaps because the increase in the mean age of the women concerned offsets it.

Table 4.15. Rate of Intrauterine Mortality at Rank n, in the Absence of Miscarriages from Ranks 1 to $n - 1$

$n = 1$	103/1,051 = 9.8%
$n = 2$	72/ 824 = 8.7%
$n = 3$	64/ 654 = 9.8%
$n = 4$	40/ 506 = 7.9%
$n = 5$	30/ 385 = 7.8%
$n = 6$	21/ 286 = 7.4%
All	330/3,706 = 8.9%

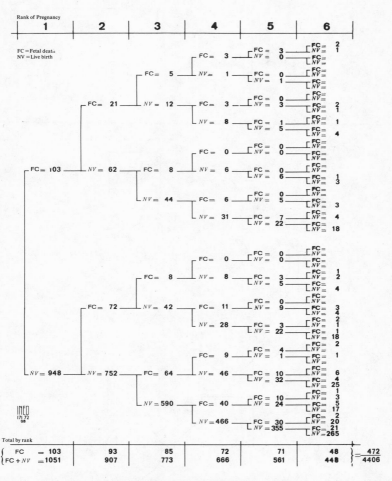

Fig. 4.2. Outcomes of successive pregnancies, for orders 1 to 6 (Martinique).

Once a first miscarriage has occurred, the risk at later ranks is about 20%, whatever the rank at which this first miscarriage occurs (see table 4.16).

After a second miscarriage, the risk is about 25% (37/144 = 25.7%); after a third, it is apparently even higher (13/23 = 56.5%).

Finally, I have attempted to find a "cluster effect" by calculating the risks at successive ranks after a first miscarriage. After regrouping results derived for each rank at which the first miscarriage occurs, we obtain table 4.17.

The risk *immediately* after the first miscarriage (20.5%) is only slightly

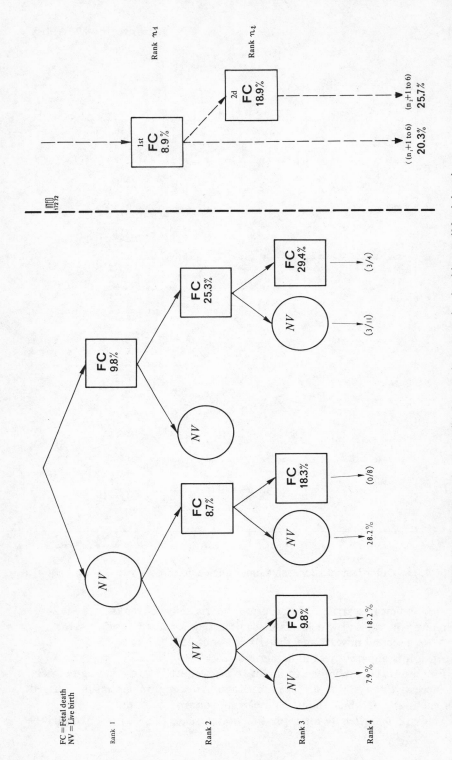

Fig. 4.3. Intrauterine mortality by previous reproductive history (Martinique).

Table 4.16. Rate of Intrauterine Mortality after a First Miscarriage Occurring at Rank n

n	Miscarriages	Live Births	Total	Rate
1	62	241	303	20.5%
2	32	143	175	18.3%
3	30	110	140	21.4%
4	16	44	60⎫	21.7%
5	2	20	22⎭	
All	142	558	700	

The header "Pregnancies of Ranks $(n + 1)$ to 6" spans the Miscarriages, Live Births, and Total columns.

different from the *overall* risk after this first miscarriage (20.3%). Examining the pregnancies occurring after second and subsequent miscarriages, we find a risk of mortality immediately after a miscarriage (whatever its rank) equal to 22.1% (73/330).

Heterogeneous Intrauterine Mortality

Similar data from a sample in Créteil are published elsewhere (Leridon 1976, ref. 142), and these data were used in estimating the distribution of the risk of intrauterine mortality among women. Positing that this risk is distributed according to a beta function, with parameters a and b (see chap. 3 for the characteristics of the beta function), we find that the probability of an ith abortion during the jth pregnancy, given that $i - 1$ abortions occurred in the previous $j - 1$ pregnancies, is:

$$Q(i, j) = \frac{a + i - 1}{a + b + j - 1}.$$

Let p be the risk of intrauterine mortality, distributed among women according to a beta function and constant for each woman. Setting the size of

Table 4.17. Rates of Intrauterine Mortality at Rank $(n + x)$ When the First Miscarriage Occurred at Rank n

Rank	Rate	
$(n + 1)$	50/244	= 20.5%
$(n + 2)$	44/189	= 23.3%
$(n + 3)$	25/138	= 18.1%
$(n + 4)$	18/ 89⎫	= 17.8%
$(n + 5)$	5/ 40⎭	
Total	142/700	= 20.3%

the cohort equal to unity, the number of women who have i abortions in j pregnancies, with a *given sequence* of pregnancy outcomes, is:

$$A(i,j) = \int_0^1 p^i(1-p)^{j-1}f(p)dp \quad (j \geq 1, \quad 0 \leq i \leq j).$$

The number of different sequences for these women is $\binom{i}{j}$.

In order for the ith abortion to occur during the jth pregnancy, the woman must have had $(i-1)$ abortions among her $(j-1)$ previous pregnancies, which is again possible in $\binom{i-1}{j-1}$ different ways. Hence:

$$Q(i,j) = \frac{A(i,j)}{A(i-1,j-1)} \quad (1 \leq i \leq j).$$

Using the expressions of $f(p)$ (as a beta function) that were given in chapter 3, we can develop $A(i,j)$ and $A(i-1,j-1)$, and we come to:

$$A(i,j) = \frac{a(a+1)\cdots(a+i-1)b(b+1)\cdots(b+j-i-1)}{(a+b)(a+b+1)\cdots(a+b+j-1)}$$

and

$$Q(i,j) = \frac{a+i-1}{a+b+j-1}.$$

It is thus possible to find the parameters a and b which best fit the data, either the distributions of figure 4.2 or the rates of figure 4.3. Without coming to a perfect fit, it is nonetheless possible to arrive at estimates which show that the hypothesis of heterogeneity is sufficient for explaining most of the results given in the preceding section, independent of the age effect.

In the case of Martinique, for an average risk of 10%, the estimated variance is 0.0073 and the parameters of the beta function are: $\hat{a} = 1.1$ $\hat{b} = 10.1$.

In table 4.18 I have compared the date given in figure 4.2 for orders 1 to 4 with the results of the model (in the model, the total number of pregnancies for each rank was set equal to the observed number of pregnancies for the same rank). There are still some discrepancies between theoretical and actual values, but as a whole the model does explain a substantial part of the data.

Pregnancy Progression Rates as a Function of Pregnancy Outcome

In the same article I have also studied the possible consequences of "pregnancy progression rates" (i.e., the probability of having another pregnancy), which differ according to the outcome of the preceding pregnancy. Some authors have suggested that the increase in the risk of intrauterine mortality with pregnancy rank or mother's age could result—at least in part—from the fact that women with high risk form a large proportion of high-rank preg-

Table 4.18. Outcome of Successive Pregnancies: Comparison between Observed Values and Model's Values (Martinique)

Pregnancy Order			
1	2	3	4
SA = 103.2(103)	SA = 15.3 (21)	SA = 3.1 (5)	SA = 0.8 (3)
			LB = 1.9 (1)
		LB = 10.0 (12)	SA = 1.9 (3)
			LB = 6.7 (8)
	LB = 73.7 (62)	SA = 10.0 (8)	SA = 1.9 (0)
			LB = 6.7 (6)
		LB = 52.8 (44)	SA = 6.7 (6)
			LB = 38.8 (31)
LB = 947.8(948)	SA = 73.8 (72)	SA = 10.0 (8)	SA = 1.9 (0)
			LB = 6.7 (8)
		LB = 52.8 (42)	SA = 6.7 (11)
			LB = 38.8 (28)
	LB = 744.2(752)	SA = 52.9 (64)	SA = 6.7 (9)
			LB = 38.8 (46)
		LB = 581.4(590)	SA = 38.8 (40)
			LB = 462.1(466)
Total: 1,051	907	773	666
% SA: Model 9.82	9.82	9.82	9.82
Observed 9.80	10.25	11.00	10.81

NOTE: Observed values are in parentheses. SA = spontaneous abortion; LB = live birth.

nancies, since women with low risk reach their desired number of children more rapidly. As a matter of fact, among couples practicing highly effective contraception there is some evidence that pregnancy progression rates are higher after a miscarriage than after a live birth, as the above hypothesis indicates. But the *opposite* result was found in the Martinique sample, at least for the first six ranks.

In any case, the scheme developed above for estimating the distribution of the risk of intrauterine mortality would have to be modified only if the continuation rates were affected by the pregnancy rank *as well as* by the outcome of the preceding pregnancy. Up to now, however, there is no evidence that these conditions hold.

We may thus consider the distribution of risk among women to be the most important factor in the analysis of intrauterine mortality and to be responsible for most of the effect of progressive selection.

To Sum Up

What can we conclude from these results? First, let us note, as Warburton and Frazer have already done, that no simple model allows us to account for all observed phenomena. On the whole, it seems true that:

1. The risk of intrauterine mortality is quite heterogeneous among individuals. This may be explained by positing either a regular distribution of risk among women (according to a beta function) or a higher mean risk for a certain proportion of women (say, 10%).

2. The risk increases with age, at least from 30–35 years on, irrespective of the previous retrospective history; this is especially true for the first pregnancy. However, the rate of increase is sometimes altered by the method of observation.

3. The presence of induced abortions that are reported as spontaneous abortions may disturb the observations. In particular, this could result in an exaggeration of the risk of repeat abortions, and thus in the variance of the risk of intrauterine mortality among women.

4. About 25% of the pregnancies in progress after 4 weeks of gestation (since the last menstrual period) end in an intrauterine death. However, this estimate can be obtained only by means of a "life table of intrauterine mortality," since rates obtained by purely retrospective data are usually on the order of 12% to 15%.

5. Except in extreme situations, it is very difficult to say whether the different rates of intrauterine mortality obtained in various populations reflect real differences in the risk for the populations or whether they are simply a result of differences in the method of observation or in the statements of the women interviewed.

Etiology of Intrauterine Mortality

This topic is principally a medical one and will be developed only briefly here. It is interesting to note, however, how much the improvement in our knowledge of the rate of occurrence of intrauterine mortality has affected the evolution of ideas on the causes of this mortality. As it has become progressively clear that most intrauterine mortality occurs during the very first weeks of gestational development, and that there may be quite a delay (i.e., several weeks) between the end of the embryo's development and its actual expulsion, explanations due to immediate causes—physical or psychological traumas undergone by the woman—have been abandoned. These events may provoke the expulsion of an embryo that is already dead, but they are rarely the cause of the death.

It is useful in general to distinguish between *late abortions* (after the 20th week) and *early abortions* (before the 20th week). More than half of the former seem to be caused by inflamed lesions, often of infectious origin. Malformations of the uterus may also play a substantial role, especially in the case of repeated miscarriages.

The etiology of early abortions is very different. Most of these are caused by anomalies in the genetic structure of the zygote, which may be of two types: anomalies affecting only one or a few genes, which may be inherited or caused by a mutation, and chromosomal anomalies, completely affecting one or several chromosomes; these are serious, and most are never seen in infants carried to term.

It is these chromosomal anomalies or "aberrations" that explain the majority of early intrauterine deaths. This has long been suspected, since the fundamental work of Hertig et al. (see ref. 1973), but further confirmation has been made possible by the systematic determination of the karyotypes (i.e., the chromosomal structure) of spontaneously aborted embryos, carried out on a large scale by D. Carr in Canada and by J. and A. Boué in France (see section 1.121 of the Bibliography). According to the observations of the latter, *nearly two-thirds* of all spontaneous abortions are due to chromosomal aberrations. Combining these results with those of Shapiro (for the overall evolution of intrauterine mortality with age) and of French and Bierman (for the general level), we have been able to decompose rates by age or pregnancy rank (Leridon and Boué 1971, ref. 181). Table 4.19 gives these results, which show that the increase in intrauterine mortality with mother's age (or pregnancy rank) is, for the most part, due to the increase in genetic risk.

Table 4.19.   Intrauterine Mortality from Genetic Causes by Age of Mother and Rank of Pregnancy

	Age of Mother					
	< 20 Years	20–24	25–29	30–34	35–39	≥ 40 Years
Overall rate per 1,000 pregnancies[a]	(207)	162	192	261	366	(500)
Proportion of Chromosomal anomalies[b]	(0.42)	0.59	0.58	0.65	0.74	0.85
Decomposition of the rate						
Chromosomal origin	(87)	96	111	170	270	(425)
Nonchromosomal origin	(120)	66	81	91	96	(75)

	Rank of Pregnancy			
	1	2	3	4 and over
Overall rate per 1,000 pregnancies[a]	162	179	230	311
Proportion of chromosomal anomalies[b]	0.58	0.65	0.65	0.66
Decomposition of the rate				
Chromosomal origin	94	116	149	205
Nonchromosomal origin	68	63	81	106

[a] 1.67 times the crude rates recorded by Shapiro et al. (ref. 151). The coefficient 1.67 is the ratio of the overall rate of the French and Bierman table (ref. 133) to the overall rate obtained by Shapiro.
[b] Based on results of Boué and Boué (see ref. 181).

In the current state of these observations it is not possible to specify in great detail the respective roles of chromosomal aberrations and other anomalies in the risk of mortality as a function of the outcomes of previous pregnancies, or as a function of the causes of previous miscarriages. This would imply a detailed discussion of the various types of anomalies and taking into account both the parents' genetic histories and the anomalies observed in infants carried to term. (See Shapiro and Abramowicz 1969, ref. 150; Boué and Boué, 1973, ref. 163.)

Toward a Complete Life Table of Intrauterine Mortality

We have already stated that the rate obtained by French and Bierman for the period 4–7 weeks is perhaps underestimated and that the actual rate might well be as high as 150 per 1,000, according to their table.

And what happens during the first two weeks of pregnancy, between ovulation and the time of the next menstrual period? Although no definitive answer can be given yet, let us try to follow the process step by step.

If fertilization has actually taken place, the result is the formation of an egg, which immediately but slowly begins its cellular division. At the time it enters the uterine cavity, about the 4th day, the egg has only about a dozen cells (when developing normally); at the end of the first week nidation has taken place, but the egg is still less than 1 mm in diameter. Expulsion of the egg may occur during the 2d or 3d week (i.e., at the time of the next menstrual period), but it is extremely difficult to distinguish a period with a fertilized egg from a normal ovulatory cycle. Theoretically, the distinction is not impossible: for example, from the very beginning of pregnancy, certain hormonal balances undergo considerable changes. However, it may be a problem in these very hormonal secretions which causes the end of development and the expulsion of the embryo. In other words, the means for detecting—even very early— a *normal* pregnancy may be invalid in the case of an *abnormal* pregnancy.

As for direct observation of the egg, its obvious consequence is an immediate end to development! However, it is by this route that some idea about the first 2 weeks of gestation has been obtained. Some very detailed work was carried out by Hertig and his associates (Hertig et al. 1949 and 1959, refs. 174 and 175) dealing with women undergoing operations (hysterectomies) that would result in permanent sterility. Because of this inevitable result, it was possible to ask the women involved to voluntarily expose themselves to optimal conditions of fertilization just before the operation. Hertig could thus (progressively) construct a small sample of women: who had already been proved fertile; who had ovulated normally during the last cycle; who had had sexual intercourse at least once less than 24 hours before or after the day of ovulation; and whose operation was not justified on the basis of some pathological state which could prevent fertilization.

Operating on these women during the days after ovulation, Hertig could try to distinguish the cases when fertilization had occurred, the egg's stage of development in those cases, and the normal or abnormal character of the egg's evolution. Out of 107 cases, he found 34 eggs that had been fertilized and were between 2 and 17 days old; 10 of these 34 were clearly abnormal. Hertig then constructed a subsample of 36 women, keeping only the cases that were done under the best possible research conditions (this is the subsample generally cited in the literature). In this group fertilization had occurred in 21 cases, of which 6 were abnormal eggs. In other words, the recognizable fecundability of this sample rose to $15/36 = 0.42$.

In 1967 Hertig wrote an excellent summary of his work and his conclusions (ref. 173). He estimates that, out of 100 ova which are brought into contact with sperm, there would be:

16 cases of nonfertilization,

15 deaths before implantation (i.e., during the 1st week),

27 deaths during the 2d week,

 8 deaths between the 3d and 6th weeks,

 3 deaths in the following months, and

31 live births (including about 1 child with congenital anomalies).

Thus, out of 42 pregnancies still in progress at the beginning of the 3d week, 11 would end in miscarriages—this rate of 26% is compatible with the findings of French and Bierman. But we must now add an equal number of pregnancies (42) terminated before the end of the 2d week.

More recently, James has reanalyzed Hertig's data and proposed somewhat different conclusions (1970, ref. 140). According to James, one will find.

that 10% of the eggs fail to be fertilized,

that 50% of the fertilized eggs are abnormal,

that 60% of these abnormal eggs disappear before the 25th day, and

that 10% of the normal eggs disappear before the 25th day.

Out of 90 fertilized eggs, there will thus be $1/2 \times 90 \times 0.6 = 27$ deaths of abnormal zygotes during the first two weeks or so; and $1/2 \times 90 \times 0.1 \simeq 5$ deaths of normal zygotes during the same period, which would leave 58 pregnancies in progress 2 weeks after fertilization. James applies the overall rate of mortality from the French and Bierman table to these 58 "survivors" and obtains $58 \times 0.237 \simeq 14$ deaths after 2 weeks, which leaves 44 live births (instead of Hertig's 31).

However, one objection to this calculation is that the proportion of abnormal zygotes which develop to full term would be much too high. That is, after 2 weeks of development, there would be $45 - 27 = 18$ abnormal zygotes, and thus, after 38 weeks of development, there would be *at least*: $18 - 14 = 4$ abnormal births out of 44 live births, or about 10%. The usual estimate for all congenital malformations, even benign ones, is less than 5%, and for chromosomal anomalies alone is around 1%.

It would not be enough to increase mortality slightly after 2 weeks, and thus include the 3 or 4 "extra" abnormal embryos, to resolve this problem, since it is unlikely that *all* the embryos dying after 2 weeks would be malformed. To convince ourselves, we may restate the problem in the following way:

Starting with the 40 normal and 18 abnormal embryos which are still developing after 2 weeks in James's scheme, we posit that at most 1 of these 18 will be carried to term. There would then be 17 spontaneously aborted abnormal embryos.

"Abnormal" embryos here means having serious anomalies, in most cases originating in the chromosomes. Since, according to J. and A. Boué, about 60% of all spontaneous abortions after 2 weeks have chromosomal anomalies, we must add to the 17 abnormal embryos $17 \times 40/60 \simeq 11$ normal embryos that are spontaneously aborted.

In all, then, there would only be $58 - 17 - 11 \simeq 30$ live-born infants. This result is nearly the same as Hertig's, but the mortality after 2 weeks is *double* the figure of French and Bierman ($28/58 \simeq 0.483$). James's schema thus seems less plausible, and Hertig's estimate seems more reliable.

Combining Hertig's results with those of French and Bierman results in the "Complete Table of Intrauterine Mortality" (see table 4.20), which includes the cases of nonfertilized ova (under optimal conditions for fertilization as mentioned above; i.e., sexual intercourse within 24 hours of ovulation).

Fecundability and Intrauterine Mortality

It is useful to return briefly to the notion of fecundability, which has so far been left out of the discussion of intrauterine mortality These two components are highly interrelated, as Henry has shown in an important article (1964, ref. 134).

According to table 4.20, "physiological" fecundability may be as high as 0.84 (and even 0.90, according to James). In fact, since the 42 spontaneous abortions of the first 2 weeks are completely unnoticed, it is possible to reduce this value immediately to 0.42, as an estimate of "recognizable" fecundability. There is no problem in doing this, *if* the risk of fertilization during each cycle is not affected by a very brief pregnancy during the previous cycle (in other words, if there is no additional nonsusceptible period). If this is true, then it is the same as saying that there had been no fertilization, or that fertilization took place but without any effect on the following cycle.

In reality, we do not know if this is true. We do know, however, that if such a conception is followed by a nonsusceptible period, it is certainly a brief one. Potter (1963, ref. 031) and Henry (1964, ref. 134) have shown that after a

Table 4.20. Complete Table of Intrauterine Mortality, per 100 Ova Exposed to
the Risk of Fertilization

Week after Ovulation x	Deaths[a] d_x	Survivors[b] S_x
	16[c]	100
0	15	84
1	27	69
2	5.0	42
6	2.9	37
10	1.7	34.1
14	0.5	32.4
18	0.3	31.9
22	0.1	31.6
26	0.1	31.5
30	0.1	31.4
34	0.1	31.3
38	0.2	31.2
Live births.		31

SOURCE: Based on results of Hertig (1967,
ref. 173) and French and Bierman (1962,
ref. 133).
[a] More precisely, expulsions of dead embryos.
[b] That is, pregnancies still in progress.
[c] Not fertilized.

miscarriage occurring during month 2 or 3 the nonsusceptible period would generally be no more than a month longer than the duration of gestation. Thus, the error possible from including intrauterine mortality of the first 2 weeks with fecundability is certainly quite small.

However, the estimate of recognizable fecundability given above (0.42) is still high. The resulting "effective fecundability," in terms of live births, would be 0.31, though I have suggested above a value of about 0.25 (at about 25 years). But we must not forget that Hertig worked with "optimal" conditions, considering only cases where there had been sexual intercourse within 24 hours of ovulation. For this to be true, for example, in a sample of newly married couples, there would have to be a (uniform) frequency of intercourse equal to once every other day, which is higher than the findings of most surveys; according to the study by Barrett and Marshall, discussed in chapter 3, recognizable fecundability would be 0.43 for this frequency, 0.31 for one intercourse every 3 days, and 0.24 for one intercourse every 4 days.

These various approaches are thus consistent in terms of *recognizable* fecundability, but not in terms of *physiological* fecundability and of the ratio between the two. However, this is not very important from the demographer's point of view, since we are usually interested in recognizable fecundability (and intrauterine mortality) only.

5

The Non-susceptible Period

Every conception, whatever its outcome, marks the beginning of a period during which fecundability is zero, a period which lasts at least as long as the pregnancy (and often much longer) and is called the nonsusceptible period.

Although daily experience has long shown that the woman is not fully fecund during the postpartum period, especially while breast-feeding, scientific and statistical data have long been lacking. Most of our knowledge on the subject comes from strictly demographic observations—that is, through birth intervals—even though the duration of postpartum amenorrhea is not always known exactly. The discussion here, however, will begin with the physiological variables and then move on to examine how the study of birth intervals provides indirect proof of the existence of a postpartum non-susceptible period. Finally, physiological data will be used in discussing the differences between populations.

Postpartum Amenorrhea and Breast-feeding

A distinction must be made at the outset of this discussion between populations with little or no breast-feeding (e.g., most of the developed Western countries) and populations where breast-feeding is prolonged and widespread. From a medical, nutritional, and sociological point of view, the distance between the two groups is too great to permit direct extrapolations from one to the other.

a. Three careful studies dealing with countries with short breast-feeding will be used here, one by Salber, Feinleib, and MacMahon in Boston (1966, ref. 225), another by Pascal in Cambrai and Paris (1969, ref. 219), which includes a complete review of the literature on the subject, and a third by Perez et al. in Santiago, Chile (1971, ref. 221). In all three cases the survey was conducted on women who had recently given birth, and for whom the following facts were recorded: (1) the duration of amenorrhea and the duration of breast-feeding (partial or full); (2) in Cambrai, the duration of anovulation, by the temperature method; (3) in Santiago, the duration of anovulation by the same method, in combination with endometrial biopsies.

In Boston, 78% of the women studied did not breast-feed at all. This proportion is smaller in the second and third samples (38% and 15% respectively), which may be more subject to selection in this respect. For these women, the mean duration of amenorrhea is 58 days in the first two samples and 69 days in the third. Since the first ovulation may occur before the return of menstruation, we see that the total nonsusceptible period does not exceed 10 to 11 months when there is no breast-feeding.

Table 5.1. Duration of Amenorrhea by Total Duration of Breast-feeding (Partial and Full Nursing; Short Durations of Breast-feeding)

Duration of Breast-feeding	Duration of Amenorrhea (in Days)				
	France[a]		Boston[b]		Santiago[c]
	Mean	Median	Mean	Median	Mean
No breast-feeding	58	52.5	58	55	44.3
Less than 1 month	52	49		56	53
1 to 2 months	68	64		68	71
2 to 3 months	82	83		85	89
3 to 4 months	95	101		112	107
4 to 5 months	115	123		124	125
5 to 6 months	126	118		155	143
Over 6 months[d]	175	(185)		(150)	...

[a] Pascal (1969, ref. 219): 425 women who breast-fed, 276 who did not.
[b] Salber et al. (1966, ref. 225): 485 women who breast-fed, 1,712 who did not.
[c] Perez et al. (1971, ref. 221): 170 women who breast-fed and 30 who did not; results adjusted by the authors.
[d] On the average, approximately 8 months.

But the duration of amenorrhea increases greatly with the duration of breast-feeding, although at a slower rate, as table 5.1 shows. The duration of breast-feeding taken into account here includes partial breast-feeding when it occurs. Up to 3 months of breast-feeding, the mean (or median) duration of amenorrhea is greater; beyond 3 months, duration of amenorrhea is shorter than that of breast-feeding. The mean duration of amenorrhea is about 4 months for a duration of breast-feeding of between 5 and 6 months.

Thus it is certain that a large proportion of women who breast-feed experience the end of amenorrhea *before* the weaning of their child (about two-thirds of those who breast-feed for at least 4 months). And the first ovulation may even *precede* the first menses: this is the most frequent case, contrary to the conclusions of earlier works, reviewed by Tietze in 1961 (ref. 229). For example, according to the study by Pascal, the first ovulation took place:

in 57% of the cases before the return of menses,
in 33% of the cases during the 1st cycle that followed,
in 6% of the cases during the 2d cycle that followed,
in 3% of the cases during the 3d cycle that followed,
in 1% of the cases during the 4th cycle that followed.

There are no significant differences by duration of breast-feeding, age, or parity.

These results are confirmed by the study of Perez et al. (78% have ovulation before the return of menses); however, in their study, the frequency was sensitive to lactation status at the time of return of ovulation.

On the average, then, it does not seem necessary to systematically add one or two supposedly anovulatory cycles onto the duration of amenorrhea, as some authors have suggested (although it is still possible for such cycles to occur at any time during fecund periods).

Nevertheless, the return to normal fecundity is probably not immediate. The first cycles are actually often irregular, and their variance much higher than normal. Here (again according to Pascal) is the evolution of the variance of successive cycles (measured in days):

$V = 48.5$ for the 1st cycle after the return of menses,
$V = 32.7$ for the 2d cycle after the return of menses,
$V = 20.2$ for the 3d cycle after the return of menses,
$V = 21.1$ for the 4th cycle after the return of menses,
$V = 15.7$ for the 5th cycle after the return of menses.

At the same time, the frequency of anovulatory cycles falls from 10% to less than 5%.

b. We have less detailed information about the situation in countries where long breast-feeding is general rule (and where the inability to breast-feed may mean the death of the infant). But there is evidence of a strong and significant correlation between duration of breast-feeding and duration of amenorrhea. This correlation has been shown directly in several studies, carried out mainly in Asia and sub-Saharan Africa; some results are shown in table 5.2 and figure 5.1.

Although the (mean or median) duration of breast-feeding may be as long as 2 years, the (mean or median) duration of amenorrhea is never longer than one and a half years. The longest durations of amenorrhea were observed in the Bangladesh (Matlab) Study: 17 months; in South Korea: 14 months; and in Senegal: about 13 months. Everywhere else the mean values are less than one year. It is thus probable that breast-feeding's inhibiting effect on ovulation weakens progressively as the period of breast-feeding increases; we will see the reasons for this further on.

On the average, the results cited above lead to the conclusion that the

Table 5.2. Mean or Median Duration of Amenorrhea by Total Duration of Breast-feeding (Long Durations of Breast-feeding)

Place	Source	Duration of Breast-feeding (Months)		Duration of Amenorrhea (Months)	
		Mean	Median	Mean	Median
Bombay	Baxi (1957; ref. 205)	16.5		11.9	
Punjab	Potter et al. (1965; ref. 224)		21		11
Bangladesh	Chen et al. (1974; ref. 024)		24[a]		17
Taiwan	Jain et al. (1970; ref. 212)	15.0	13.8	10.1	11.4
South Korea	Koh and Smith (1970; ref. 217	24		14.6	14
Thailand[c]	Sivin (1974; ref. 369)	11.2		6.1	
Rwanda	Bonte and Van Balen (1969; ref. 207)		18		12
Senegal	Cantrelle and Leridon (1971; ref. 208)	24.3	24	15[b]	13[b]
Dakar	Ferry (1976; ref. 328*b*)	18.9	17.6	9.8	7.9
Turkey, Iran[d]	Sivin (1974; ref. 369)	13.0		6.2	
Colombia, Venezuela[e]	Sivin (1974; ref. 369)	7.6		3.9	

[a] In the case of conception during breast-feeding, the duration is counted only until the conception. The true duration is probably greater than 25 months.
[b] Indirect estimate.
[c] Four countries in Southeast Asia—72% from Thailand.
[d] Three countries in west Asia—90% women from Turkey and Iran.
[e] Four countries in Latin America—71% women from Colombia and Venezuela.

total nonsusceptible period (for a live birth) is a minimum of around 20 months when breast-feeding is widespread and prolonged. We shall now confirm these results by indirect methods.

Birth Intervals

The existence of a nonsusceptible period that widely exceeds the duration of gestation is proved, as I have said, by the fact that intervals between births are, on the average, distinctly longer than the interval between marriage and first birth. The former have been given as about 24 months (at 20–25 years, i.e., early in marriage), and the latter as 14 months: a difference of *10 months* which cannot be attributed to chance. (Some data of this type are given in table 5.3.)

Let us leave aside for the moment the problem of intrauterine mortality. The duration of gestation varies little, and so knowledge of the interval between two births allows us to calculate the sum: postpartum nonsusceptible period + mean time to conception.

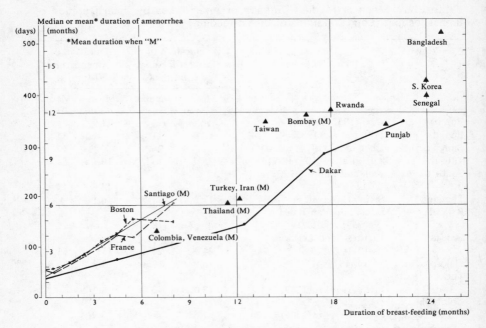

Fig. 5.1. Median (or mean) duration of amenorrhea by total duration of breast-feeding.

Thus, there are two distinct sources of variability to consider when comparing intervals to study their variation with age or to estimate differences among individuals. Henry has studied the problems posed by this interrelationship (1964, ref. 210) and proposed two conclusions:

1. the comparisons between intervals from marriage to first birth and intervals between births give a good estimate of the length of the nonsusceptible period (despite the discontinuity that could be introduced by the first pregnancy);

2. the nonsusceptible period seems to increase with age, over 30 years, as fecundability is decreasing.

In addition, the existence of intrauterine mortality does not disturb this schema.

D'Souza (1973, ref. 027a) has proposed a method for simultaneously estimating fecundability and the nonsusceptible period, using the distribution of birth intervals. His model posits a mean time to conception (for a live birth) of the form

$$e^{-\alpha t}\left(\text{mean } \frac{1}{\alpha}, \quad \text{variance } \frac{1}{\alpha^2}\right)$$

Table 5.3. Birth Intervals and the Nonsusceptible Period

Type of Interval	Quebec	Crulai	Ile-de-France	Mean Intervals in Months Tunis	Tourouvre-au-Perche	Senegal	Mommlingen	Taiwan[d]
Marriage–first birth[a]	17.3	16.3[b]	14.2		17.3[b]			
First–second birth	22.5	26.5[b]	22.8		24.5[b]			
Fate of the infant born at the beginning of the interval								
dead before 6 months	18.8	⎱20.7[c]	20.6	18.4	⎱20.7[c]			
dead between 6 and 12 months	23.5	⎰	26.4	23.2	⎰			
survived to 1 year	25.0	29.6[c]	27.2	27.5	30.0[c]			
dead between 0 and 3 months						19.7	16.1[e]	
dead between 3 and 6 months						21.5	17.0[f]	
dead between 6 and 9 months						22.1	⎱20.2	⎱11.4(+9)
dead between 9 and 12 months						25.1	⎰	⎰
survived to 1 year						32.7	27.5	17.3(+9)
survived to 3½ years						33.7	—	—

SOURCES: Quebec: Henripin (1954, ref. 335); Crulai: Gautier and Henry (1958, ref. 332); Ile-de-France: Ganiage (1963, ref. 331); Tourouvre: Charbonneau (1970, ref. 323); Senegal: Cantrelle and Leridon (1973, ref. 208); Mommlingen: Knodel (1970, ref. 346); Taiwan: Jain (1969, ref. 211); Tunis: Ganiage (1960, ref. 330).

[a] Births beginning at eight months of marriage only.
[b] Women married between 20 and 30 years of age.
[c] Means of the mean intervals of each type, per family, not weighted (families of size 3 to 13).
[d] Interval calculated from birth to next conception (add 9 months for comparison with other figures).
[e] Deaths between 0 and 1.2 months.
[f] Deaths between 1.2 and 6 months.

and a nonsusceptible period distributed normally (with mean μ and variance σ^2). Under these conditions, the distribution of intervals between live births will have the following characteristics:

$$\text{mean: } \mu + \frac{1}{\alpha}$$

$$\text{variance: } \sigma^2 + \frac{1}{\alpha^2}$$

$$\text{third-order moment: } \frac{2}{\alpha^3}$$

The parameters α, μ, and σ^2 are estimated from observed moments, by the method of maximum likelihood.

Actually, the method is of limited interest in estimating fecundability, since, even if the estimation of the mean time to conception is correct, the main problem is to derive from it the mean fecundability. D'Souza simply takes the reciprocal of the time to conception, which gives a systematically low estimate if fecundability is not homogeneous; as we have seen in chapter 3, the inverse of the mean time to conception is equal to the *harmonic* mean of fecundabilities, which can be quite different from the arithmetic mean. However, the method gives a direct estimate of the mean and variance of the nonsusceptible period which seems satisfactory, although the choice of a symmetrical distribution (normal distribution) may be criticized.

Another idea is to examine the *increase* in the nonsusceptible period resulting from breast-feeding by grouping intervals according to the age at death of the infant born at the beginning of the interval.

One consequence of the death of an infant is an immediate end to breast-feeding and thus also an end to the inhibition of ovulation due to breast-feeding. Many monographs in historical demography propose such comparisons between intervals "after death" (for an infant dying before 6 months or before 1 year of life) and intervals "without death" (infant still alive after 1 year); the means of the intervals may be calculated in various ways (means by rank, by family, weighted or nonweighted, etc.). Table 5.3 shows several results: the differences run from 6 months to 10 months, when comparing the case of an infant dying before 6 months with the case where he survives at least 1 year.

The total number of women included in each monograph is small, so the calculation has not generally been done in a detailed way (except by Knodel, for Mommlingen in Bavaria). A follow-up survey, carried out by Cantrelle in Senegal, has given us the chance to study the interrelations between fecundity, breast-feeding, and infant mortality more thoroughly (Cantrelle and Leridon 1971, ref. 208).

Table 5.4.   Senegal: Birth intervals, by Age at Death or Age at Weaning of the First of Two Children

Age at Death or at Weaning (in Months)	At Weaning	Mean Interval by Age At Death	At Death, for Deaths before Conception of the Second Child
0–2		19.7	19.7
3–5	25.1	21.5	22.0
6–8		22.1	22.4
9–11		25.1	25.7
12–14	25.4	26.8	28.4
15–17	28.4	30.0	31.5
18–20	28.7	30.9	34.9
21–23	32.5	28.9	33.8
24–26	34.7	31.2	38.3
27–29	37.2	33.5	40.6
30–32	37.8	33.5	(45.2)[a]
33–35	40.9	32.7	(50.0)[a]
All ages at weaning	33.4		
Death at ages 0–42 months		27.6	27.6
Child surviving to 42 months		33.7	...
All intervals	30.9	30.9	...

SOURCE: Cantrelle and Leridon (1971, ref. 208).
[a] Less than 10 intervals.

In particular, we have been able to calculate the intervals between births by the age at weaning of the preceding child (by periods of 3 months), by the age at death of the preceding child (by periods of 3 months), and by whether the child died before or during the next pregnancy (cf. table 5.4).

In all three cases the interval increased rapidly: 12 months, on the average, when comparing an age at death of less than 3 months with an age at death of more than 18 months. (The number of cases of weaning, without death, before 1 year was too small to warrant serious analysis.) Beyond 2 years of age, the curves differ appreciably, but part of the difference results from a "truncation" effect.

Figure 5.2 shows an *approximate decomposition* of the interval. The duration of postpartum sterility (which I take to be equal to the duration of amenorrhea) is equal to the length of the interval minus the duration of gestation (9 months) and of "mean time to conception of a live-born infant." In the article cited, the effective fecundability of the group studied was estimated to be 0.18–0.19. According to the results of table 3.2, the corresponding mean time to conception would be about 8 months. Thus we can deduce the duration of postpartum sterility, which is responsible for the differences in the

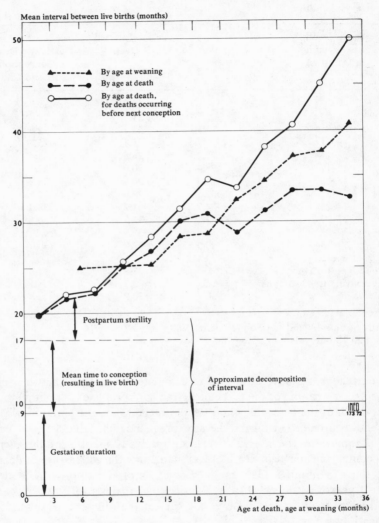

Fig. 5.2. Intervals between births by age at weaning or age at death (Senegal).

length of intervals. In table 5.5 these results are compared with the results obtained by Pascal (cf. table 5.1.).

For Senegal, I have used intervals by age at *death*, since weaning before 1 year is very rare unless the child dies. Despite the great differences between the two populations studied, the two series are quite similar; but only relatively short durations of breast-feeding are considered here.

Table 5.5. Duration of Postpartum Sterility in Two Populations, by Duration of Breast-feeding

Duration of Breast-feeding (in Months)	Duration of Post-partum Sterility (in Months)	
	Senegal (Estimation)	France[a] (Duration of Amenorrhea)
0–3	2.7	2.2
3–6	4.5	3.8
6–9	5.1	5.0
9–12	8.1	...

[a] From J. Pascal (1969, ref. 219).

Variation with Age and Variance of Intervals

Up to this point I have mentioned neither the variability of the non-susceptible period with age nor its variance within a population. The studies on these subjects are rare, and the principal references remain the study of Potter et al. in Punjab (already cited; ref. 032), and an article by Henry (1958, ref. 028).

Taking the mother's age into consideration poses a particular problem. An interval between births is not, of course, an instantaneous event for which one can determine an age without ambiguity. Thus certain conventions must be adopted. If we take the age at the beginning of the interval, there is a severe bias at the end of the reproductive period: only short intervals could be taken into account. On the other hand, if we take the age at the end of the interval, there will be a similar bias at the beginning of the reproductive period. The solution adopted by Potter et al. was to take the age at the beginning of the

Table 5.6. Punjab: Birth Intervals and Duration of Amenorrhea (in Months), by Age of the Woman

	15–19	20–24	25–29	30–34	35–39	49 and More	All Ages
Duration of Amenorrhea							
Mean[a]	7.4	9.4	10.7	12.3	12.9	13.9	10.8
Variance	30.4	57.9	40.5	47.0	77.2	99.7	55.0
Interval							
Mean		....30.5[b]....			.....35.0[c]..........		31.3
Variance		....180.4			......282.7		196.0

SOURCE: Potter et al. (1965, ref. 032).
[a] Age measured at the end of the amenorrhea.
[b] Age at the beginning of the interval (635 intervals).
[c] Age at the end of the interval (423 intervals).

interval for the younger age groups and the age at the end of the interval for the older age groups.

It seems (cf. table 5.6) that the increase in the duration of amenorrhea with age could explain about *half* of the lengthening of the intervals, with the other half resulting from the decrease in fecundability and, even more, from the increase in intrauterine mortality. Henry has obtained a similar result by indirect methods, but other studies have shown a lesser increase in the non-susceptible period with age.

The analysis of variance of the intervals may be done in two ways: either by determining the portion explained by each component of the interval (nonsusceptible period, time to conception, intrauterine mortality), or by studying the variances within and between families.

Using the second approach, Henry (1958) has shown that: (1) the major part of the variance is between families; (2) most of the intrafamilial variance results from the random nature of the reproductive process.

In other words, there are "long-interval" families and "short-interval" families. For a given mean interval, the variances differ mainly because of this randomness. The importance of this "random component" is also shown in the study of Potter et al., where the authors conclude that only a quarter of the variance of the birth intervals is explained by the variance of the non-susceptible period.

Differences between Populations

In presenting the results of table 5.1 and 5.2, I emphasized the importance of the duration of breast-feeding as a determinant of the duration of amenorrhea. However, even with an equal duration of breast-feeding, the duration of amenorrhea may not always be the same: this does in fact appear in table 5.2 and figure 5.1.

One reason is that we have considered the *total* duration of breast-feeding, whether full or partial. But we know from various observations and from research on the physiology of breast-feeding that the end of amenorrhea is accelerated by the change to mixed feeding of the infant. This change may take place at different ages depending on the country or the region, and these differences were not considered above.

The sterilizing effect of breast-feeding results from the secretion of certain hormones (such as prolactin) in response to the infant's sucking on the mother's breast (cf. Jelliffe and Jelliffe 1972, ref. 214; Buchanan 1975, ref. 207b). Thus if this sucking slackens (for example, because the infant is eating other foods), the duration of amenorrhea will be shortened. On the other hand, if the sucking is more energetic (for example, in the absence of other foods or because the mother's milk is of poor quality), amenorrhea will be prolonged.

Hence it is quite probable that the correspondence between duration of breast-feeding and duration of amenorrhea is not exact: the effect of breast-feeding will be more or less intensive depending on local circumstances (nutrition, epidemiology, climate, etc.). In other words, looking again at figure 5.1, the dispersion of the points for long breast-feeding could be due to the fact that there are different relationships in different countries; for short breast-feeding, the relationship between breast-feeding and amenorrhea is apparently quite similar among various countries, probably because nearly all the countries involved have a high level of nutrition.

Ginsberg (1973, ref. 209) has proposed a model to take these points into account, in which the duration of postpartum amenorrhea is a doubly stochastic process. He distinguishes three possible states: full nursing, partial nursing, and no nursing. In each state, the duration of anovulation is distributed according to a gamma function:

$$f(t) = \frac{\lambda(\lambda t)^{k-1}}{(k-1)!} e^{-\lambda t}$$

where λ depends on the intensity of the relation between breast-feeding and anovulation. For a given socioeconomic context, there are thus three parameters, λ_1, λ_2, and λ_3, corresponding to each of the three states mentioned above.

The time spent in each state (duration of full breast-feeding and duration of partial breast-feeding) is supposed to be distributed according to negative exponentials, with means $1/\alpha$ and $1/\beta$ respectively. These parameters are estimated directly from the observed distributions.

Ginsberg was able to verify this model for populations with short breast-feeding (Boston, Santiago). Its application to situations with long breast-feeding has not yet been fully tested, but it opens some interesting horizons.

Amenorrhea under Special Circumstances

The possible influence of nutrition on the duration of amenorrhea (or of anovulation) leads us to discuss briefly periods of amenorrhea which may occur under special circumstances. A woman may sometimes be in a non-susceptible state when she is not in a postpartum period. There are frequent reports in medical literature of cases of amenorrhea under conditions of famine or severe malnutrition (cf. Bergues 1948, ref. 206; LeRoy-Ladurie 1969, ref. 218; Stein and Susser 1975, ref. 228). Some observations were made during the Second World War in cities that were blockaded and could not obtain food (e.g., Stalingrad, cities of Holland) and in prison camps. Amenorrhea was indisputably present and was probably accompanied by anovulation.

The interesting study by Stein and Susser on cities of Holland shows a considerable drop in the birth rate 9 months after these cities had difficulties with food supplies, a drop not observed in other parts of Holland subject to the difficult conditions of war but with a better food situation. Two points are of special interest:

1. the negative correlation between nutrition and fecundity is observed only when the mean daily calorie ration falls below 1,500 calories (it had dropped to 500 calories);

2. the decline in the conception rate occurs after a lag of about 2 months, whereas the return to normal happens very quickly.

Of course it is difficult to be sure that the nutrition variable was the only cause. These results, however, are corroborated by experimental studies in progress at Harvard (Frisch 1975, ref. 040*b*, and 1974, ref. 066*b*).

Let me add that, insofar as all the reproductive functions are affected, *fecundability* could also be reduced, even in the absence of complete anovulation.

The Question of Taboos on Sexual Intercourse

There is evidence of taboos of varying severity on sexual intercourse during the postpartum period, not only in many "primitive" populations but also in many "modern" populations (including, in this latter group, populations such as those of Europe during the seventeenth and eighteenth centuries). Most often, the restriction is directly and explicitly linked to breast-feeding: while the woman is breast-feeding her child, she must avoid sexual intercourse.

The most evident rational foundation for such a custom is probably that if the woman conceived again a short time after childbirth, she would have to wean her infant too soon, which—in the absence of a substitute for the mother's milk—would threaten its very survival. Various other considerations, whether or not they are medically founded, may be added to this: for example, the risk of "spoiling the mother's milk" by sexual intercourse (even not followed by conception); of provoking the return of menses; of endangering the mother's health, and so forth (cf., for example, van de Walle and van de Walle 1972, ref. 230).

It is also possible that, at least in certain societies, there is a contraceptive purpose present: the comparison between women whose children die very young (a fairly common situation, because infant mortality is often high) and other women makes possible an empirical judgment of the effect of breast-feeding. The mean interval between births for a woman who breast-feeds a child for 2 years is about one year longer than the same interval for a woman whose child dies during its first month, a fact which even the least discerning observer could hardly fail to notice. Under these conditions, the protection of the infant (with the obligation of breast-feeding) and the contraceptive purpose (with or without sexual taboos) may be so thoroughly intertwined that it becomes impossible to separate one effect from the other.

An important point is whether practice follows theory—that is, whether the taboo which is said to exist is actually respected. The sociocultural context is fundamental here: though a suspension of intercourse lasting several months (say, from 1 to 4 months) can easily be accepted even in the absence of any compulsion, a restriction applied to the entire period of breast-feeding (1 year, 2 years, sometimes longer) would require somewhat greater prudence. This is especially true under conditions of strict monogamy; we may note, for instance, that the Catholic Church has never imposed such an obligation, although it did prohibit intercourse during pregnancy and under other circumstances. In a "natural fertility" society, if the taboo were respected completely, and if it applied at all to the period of gestation as well, then sexual intercourse would be permitted for only as long as the mean time to conception—6 or 8 months at the most out of every 2 or 3 years!

A good indicator of resumption of intercourse before weaning of the infant is the proportion of infants who are weaned during the mother's next pregnancy. In Senegal, for the sample cited above, this proportion reaches 30%, with a duration of breast-feeding of about 2 years. Since monthly fecundability is much less than 1, the proportion of couples who resume intercourse before weaning must be well over 30%.

Finally, it is evident that the sexual taboo can have an effect on fertility only if its lasts *longer* than the period of postpartum amenorrhea; so it is most likely to be respected at the time when the woman is already sterile and may well be abandoned (or followed less strictly) at the time when she becomes fertile again.

Conclusion

The essential point remains that *the general abandonment of the practice of breast-feeding has considerably reduced the duration of postpartum sterility* among women of Western countries (and elsewhere). The corresponding nonsusceptible period has fallen from an average length of 10 to 12 months (sometimes less, as in certain early European populations of the seventeenth and eighteenth centuries, where the practice of breast-feeding was limited) to less than 3 months, which reduces the mean interval between two live births from approximately 28 to 30 months to a "potential" length of just over 20 months. However, contraception has more than compensated for this potential reduction.

With the decrease in fertility and in the duration of breast-feeding, the nonsusceptible period has a smaller place in the reproductive lives of women. Salber has calculated in the article cited above, that Boston women spend, on the average, 7% of their reproductive periods (from ages 12 to 45) in a nonsusceptible state, while women of Punjab spend about 40% of their reproductive periods in that state (*total* nonsusceptible time, including periods of gestation). Other calculations showing the importance of the nonsusceptible period in determining the level of fertility will be given in chapter 7.

6 Permanent Sterility

Introduction and Definitions

Sterility, as it can be measured by demographers, is a couple's incapacity to produce a live-born child. Thus, although the border between "fecundity" and "sterility" seems fairly clear, it is not sufficient to remove all ambiguity. For example, here are the definitions given in the English and French versions of the United Nations *Multilingual Demographic Dictionary* (item 622):

> A sterile couple cannot procreate a child. The sterility may be due to either or both partners and either or both may prove to be fecund with another mate. Among women, we distinguish *primary sterility* (1) where the woman has never been able to have children, and *secondary sterility* (2) which arises after one or more children have been born.

> La stérilité d'un couple (incapacité de procréation) peut provenir de celle de l'un des deux partenaires, ou d'une incompatabilité biologique entre eux. On distingue la *stérilité totale* (1) ou incapacité de procréer aucun enfant, de la *stérilité partielle* (2), ou incapacité de procréer un nouvel enfant après en avoir déjà procréé au moins un. (Ne pas confondre la sterilité partielle avec la stérilité secondaire, expression médicale désignant une stérilité consécutive à une maladie ou à un traumatisme.)

In order to compare these two passages, we must first note that there is a peculiarity of language: the English word "fecund" is the exact equivalent of the French "fertile" (both meaning capable of procreating), and the English term "fertile" exactly signifies the French term "fécond" (both meaning "having actually reproduced").

In addition, while French makes clear antonyms of "stérile" and "fertile," and also of "infécond" and "fécond," English gives either "sterile" or "infecund" as opposites of "fecund," and "infertile" as opposite of "fertile." These differences are summarized in the accompanying table.

	French	*English*
Capacity for procreation:	fertilité	fecundity
Opposite:	infertilité	infecundity
	stérilité	sterility
Actual procreation:	fécondité	fertility
Opposite:	infécondité	infertility
Probability of conceiving during a monthly cycle:	fécondabilité	fecundability

Returning to the definitions quoted above, we find that the two dictionaries give *primary* sterility as the equivalent of "stérilité *totale*," and *secondary* sterility as the equivalent of "stérilité *partielle*." In the French edition, the expression "stérilité primaire" is not used, and the expression "stérilité secondaire" must be limited to medical usage (i.e., sterility following an illness or psychological trauma). These apparently minor differences conceal important differences in viewpoint.

Let us imagine the case of a woman who is fecund at 20 years of age and marries at age 30 a man who is also fecund. The couple does not manage to have a child. Leaving aside the question of a potential biological incompatibility between the two spouses, let us suppose that medical tests have shown the woman to be sterile. According to the English definition, this is a case of primary sterility, since the woman (or the couple) proves incapable of having a child. This conclusion applies to the age at which this incapacity is ascertained, whatever the situation might have been between 20 and 30 years of age.

According to the French definition, however, we may not be able to say that this is a case of "total sterility," since we have stated that the woman was actually fecund for some years (between age 20 and some age less than 30).

The problem lies in choosing between a "prospective" point of view (in which capacity is the key factor) and the more pragmatic "retrospective" point of view (in which one attempts to *ascertain* an unambiguous state a posteriori). Demographic observation implies the use of this latter perspective, which I shall hence maintain. This is especially true since, usually, the only pregnancies registered are those which result in live births, and so we have no knowledge of other pregnancies which could prove the woman's ability to conceive or even to procreate (in the case of a stillbirth). The terms "primary" and "total" sterility will thus both be considered as representing the situation of a couple which does not succeed in producing a live-born child.

Likewise, although the French definition clearly limits the use of the term "secondary sterility" to medical causes, these limits are not clear: for example, are consequences of childbirth to be included in "medical" causes or not? Is not childbirth itself a sort of "trauma" for the female organism? The French "partial sterility" is meant to be a broader term; however, it will be used interchangeably here with the English term "secondary sterility."

Infertility and Sterility

Since our task is defined as ascertaining cases of sterility (whether partial or total) a posteriori, my estimates will be based on observations of *infertility*. In the absence of contraception, there is a clear link between infertility and sterility. Given a group of women of age x who have just given birth, we know that all these women are fertile at age x (or, more precisely, at age x minus 9 months). A certain proportion of them (S_x) will have no more children: they will thus become sterile before having time to conceive again. In other words, S_x is an estimate of the proportion of women who become sterile between $x(- 9$ months) and $x + d$, where d is the time to conception leading to a live birth (including the postpartum nonsusceptible period).

The important point is that this interval includes a gestation and a birth: hence, the proportion S_x takes into account the risk of sterility *due to a pregnancy*. We can indeed consider two general factors involved in the risk of a fecund woman becoming sterile: her increase in age (risk of "spontaneous" or physiological sterility), and her pregnancies and childbirths, which could accidentally disturb her reproductive functions.

Vincent, in 1950 (ref. 243) and Henry, in 1953 (ref. 235) have indicated means of isolating these two factors, as we shall see here.

Primary Sterility

In a noncontracepting population, a married couple which remains child-less for some years (say, 5) may be considered *sterile*; this is primary sterility if counting the first 5 years of marriage, and secondary sterility if counting 5 years after a live birth. (In this latter case, the time period must be increased if the couple is over 35 years of age, since the delay of conception can be significantly longer.)

If newly married couples are grouped by age at marriage (usually according to the woman's age), the proportion $_xS_0$ of couples married at age x and remaining childless is an estimate of the rate of primary sterility at age $x + d$, where fertile couples married at the same age have their first child on the average. We see that $1 - S_0$ is the "zero-order parity progression ratio," usually denoted by a_0. Thus, following the various $_xS_0$ (or a_0's) is a way of following the evolution of the rate of primary sterility with age.

In reality, this estimate is valid only for *married* couples. This restriction is important if there is some reason for believing that the rate of sterility is not the same for married and single people. For example, the fact that some marriages are induced by a pregnancy which has already begun could increase the fecundity of *married* couples.

Vincent has proposed the following estimate (1950, ref. 243, table IV), based on "family statistics" of three groups of European origin (workers in the French mines, families of rural Quebec, and inhabitants of England and Wales) (table 6.1).

Table 6.1. Percentage of Sterile Couples among Newlyweds

	Approximate Age (a) of the Wife					
	21	25	30	34.5	39.5	44.5
Percentage Couples Sterile at Age a	4	6	10	16	33	69

Source: Vincent 1950, ref. 243.

Secondary Sterility

The "parity progression ratio" method may be extended to successive ages or birth orders. For example, we may use the parity progression ratio of rank 1 (a_1), of rank 2 (a_2), and so forth, to give the proportion of couples which had at least two children (of those who have had one child already), at least three children (of those who have had two), and so forth. But $1 - a_n$ is thus a measure of the *newly sterile couples* between mean age at the nth birth and mean age at the $n + 1^{st}$ birth, since all the couples were fecund at the beginning of the interval.

We may compare the evolution with age given by $(1 - a_n)$ with that given by $-\Delta a_0/a_0$, as Vincent has done in the article cited above (1950, ref. 243). Thus, $-\Delta a_0/a_0$ represents new sterility due to aging alone[1] between ages x and $x + 3$ among the a_0 couples still fertile at age x, if the difference between the mean ages at the births of the two children is three years. On the other hand, however, $(1 - a_n)$ includes the effects of childbirth as well as those of age.

The couples considered in calculating a_1, a_2, etc., have been selected by the fact that they have had at least one child. It is interesting to note, however, that whether they have had one, two, three, four, or five children is unimportant, since "the probability that a family considered at the birth of a live-born infant will increase in size is, given equal age of the women at the time of the birth, independent of the rank of the birth" (Henry 1953, ref. 235). In practice, this is true for ranks 1 to 5 but not beyond, because of the heterogeneity of fecundability.

This result is not evident a priori: it amounts to stating that *the probability of becoming newly sterile is independent of the number of children already born.* It is still true that sterility may be acquired at the time of a birth: this is why the tables of newly acquired sterility for women who are already mothers (parity progression ratios a_1, a_2, etc.) and for women who are newly married (parity progression ratio a_0) cannot be identical. But this *additional* risk is the same at each birth.

1. Actually, $(1 - a_0)$ includes the risk of sterility owing to a first pregnancy which did not result in a live birth (e.g., a miscarriage).

According to the results obtained by Vincent, the risk of new sterility for women who are already mothers seems distinctly higher than the risk due to age alone until ages 30 to 35.

Finally, then, taking into account the reservations that must always be made because of various selection biases, we find that the risk of "spontaneous" acquisition of sterility for women who have already been fertile (i.e., had at least one child) is about the same as for women still single and infertile; but at each childbirth the former group is subject to a supplementary risk, which is nearly constant.

Rate of Sterility by Age

Let us now return to the question, apparently more simple, of determining the proportion of women sterile at a given age, regardless of their marital status or previous reproductive history.

According to the previous section, we can use $1 - a_0$ as a suitable estimate for newly married women. However, there are other possible procedures.

Let us consider age group $(x, x + a)$, and assume that we know for each woman whether she has had a birth within this age-group $x, x + a$, and at an older age.

Let:

N' be the number of women giving birth between x and $x + a$ *and* at an older age,

N'' be the number of women giving birth for the last time between x and $x + a$,

N_0 be the number of women having no more children after age x,

n' be the number of births between x and $x + a$ for the first group,

n'' be the number of births between x and $x + a$ for the second group;

$N = N' + N'' + N_0$;

$n = n' + n''$.

The overall fertility rate for the age-group is

$$f = n/N.$$

The fertility rate specific to women subsequently fertile is

$$f' = n'/N'.$$

Let us now assume that fertility in age-group $(x, x + a)$ was the same for women subsequently fertile as for others:

$$\frac{n'}{N'} = \frac{n''}{N''}.$$

Hence,

$$\frac{f}{f'} = \frac{N'}{N}\frac{n}{n'} = \frac{N'}{N}\left(\frac{n' + n''}{n'}\right) = \frac{N'}{N}\left(1 + \frac{N''}{N'}\right)$$

$$\frac{f}{f'} = 1 - \frac{N_0}{N}.$$

The ratio of f to f' is thus equal to the proportion of women who were still fertile after age x. This proportion is *lower* than the proportion of women not sterile (still fecund) at age x, since, as I have previously mentioned, among women still fecund at age x, some may become sterile before having time to conceive again. The proportion of women sterile at age $x + 2.5$ is probably close to the proportion of women infertile after age x.

This method was suggested by Henry. Working with five series of fertility rates, from populations of European origin (seventeenth to nineteenth centuries), he gave the estimates shown in table 6.2 (one of the five series was established by the parity progression method).

Table 6.2.   Percentage of Sterile Married Couples by Age

	Woman's Age				
	20	25	30	35	40
% sterile	3	6	10	16	31

SOURCE: Henry 1960 (ref. 340).

This series is very close to the one cited above which was based on the zero-order parity progression ratios, a_0. But despite this similarity we must recognize that our knowledge of sterility remains very imprecise. It is based on few observations, all from historical populations; and the spread of contraception has made observations in contemporary populations nearly impossible.

Another important point is that, because of the rapid increase in the rate of sterility after age 35, the proportions of *women subsequently infertile* by age differ considerably from the series of *sterility rates* at the same ages. Table 6.3 gives the values proposed by Henry for the infertility rates corresponding to the sterility rates in table 6.2.

Table 6.3.   Percentage of Married Couples Not Fertile after a Stated Age

	Woman's Age					
	20	25	30	35	40	45
% infertile	4	8	12	20	50	95

SOURCE: Henry 1960 (ref. 340).

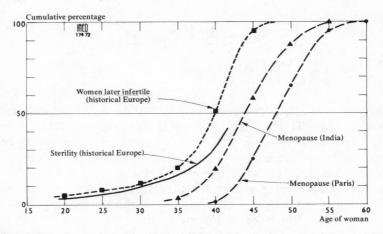

Fig. 6.1.   Proportion of women menopausal, sterile, or subsequently infertile, by age.

Finally, we compare these rates with the proportion of menopausal women by age (see fig. 6.1). Some data from table 1.2 have been used, along with the averages of two Parisian and two Indian series of rates. Of course it is difficult to know whether the women of historical Europe went through menopause at ages close to those of Parisian women today, or of Indian women today; in the second case, the proportion of menopausal women by age would give us a slightly overestimated value of the rate of sterility by age (over 40), since the two series tend to be very close after this age. But in the first case we would conclude that sterility precedes menopause by more than five years on the average.

Remaining Problems

Our knowledge on the existence and size of differentials between populations is even more limited for levels of sterility than for topics discussed in the previous chapters. Despite an inability to propose a good estimate of these differences, I can propose two arguments in favor of their existence.

First of all, if the differentials reported in chapter 1 on the progression of menopause with age are correct, we can think that they also result in differentials in the progression of sterility with age. In the models that will be described in the next chapter, I have considered three hypotheses: (1) "low" sterility, corresponding closely to the data of Vincent and Henry; (2) "high" sterility, obtained by assuming that the same rates were reached 5 years younger; and (3) an intermediate series, suggested by the fact that fertility rates obtained for ages above 35 years with the second series seemed too low.

Second, the etiology of pathological sterility leads one to believe that there could be a fairly strong link between the level of sterility and the general sanitary conditions of an area and, more precisely, endemic venereal diseases (especially gonorrhea). Romaniuk (1968, ref. 241) has cited this argument for certain populations of Zaire, and A. Retel-Laurentin (1967, ref. 240) has demonstrated it even more conclusively for the Nzakara of the Central African Republic. However, as McFalls (1973, ref. 238) emphasizes, this possibility must not become a catchall argument: it is most likely that sanitary conditions would have to be particularly bad for there to be any appreciable effect on fertility.

Finally, the problem is further complicated in modern populations by better treatment of pathological sterility and, with the opposite effect, by numerous techniques of surgical intervention which may have the effect (desired or not) of sterilizing the woman.

Yet the fact remains that a certain proportion of couples find themselves sterile before having had time to reach their desired family size, and this problem deserves more attention than it has received to date. The interested reader is referred to surveys which include some analysis of the problems of sterility and subfecundity: the "Growth of the American Family" studies (R. Freedman and others, *Family Planning, Sterility, and Population Growth* [New York: McGraw-Hill, 1959]; P. K. Whelpton and others, *Fertility and Family Planning in the United States* [Princeton: Princeton University Press, 1966]); a Belgian study (R. L. Cliquet, "The Sociobiological Aspects of the National Survey on Fecundity and Fertility in Belgium," *Journal of Biosocial Science* 1 [1969]: 369–88); and a study in New Orleans (Harter 1970, ref. 234).

Finally, a word about periods of temporary sterility is in order here. Actually, these have been discussed already to some extent, since the periods of postpartum sterility are its most common form, but it may occur at other times as well, for example, in the form of anovular cycles. Estimates on the frequency of these cycles vary between 5% and 15%; the most important point is whether they occur in clusters or singly, since in the second case (but not in the first) they may be covered in estimates of fecundability. Poor nutrition could be responsible for a higher incidence of anovular cycles.

Although my estimates are imprecise, it is certain that the spontaneous appearance of sterility before 45 or 40 years of age is an important factor in reduction of potential fertility within a cohort. With other things equal, the mean number of children per woman married at age 20 (under conditions of natural fertility) would probably increase by 35%–40% if no woman became sterile before the age of 50, and by 15%–25% if no woman became sterile before the age of 45 (I will give examples in the next chapter).

7

Levels of Natural Fertility

Introduction

Having discussed in detail each of the natural components of fertility, I shall now return to a more usual level of analysis. This will be done in two ways: first by examining available data on populations which do not practice birth control, then by comparing these data with the results of "microdemographic" models, making use of the results given in previous chapters.

Defining a "natural" level of fertility is not as simple a task as it might first appear. It even becomes a purely abstract problem when taken in the following sense: "What would the fertility be if this population did not use any method of fertility regulation?"

Such a question forces us to look for points of reference in populations in which both the following conditions obtain: (1) absence of all methods of birth control (including sterilization and induced abortion); and (2) availability of satisfactory demographic data.

For historical reasons these two conditions are often mutually exclusive and are found together in only three circumstances: (1) in contemporary populations whose fertility has not yet declined and where, in the general absence of vital records,[1] it is possible to make special surveys; (2) in late nineteenth century populations which, although they had not experienced a decline in fertility, already possessed a good registration system (Northern European countries, for example); (3) in historical populations (before the nineteenth century) which can be studied indirectly by using parish registers, genealogies, and so forth.

In the preceding chapters we have had to refer sometimes to data collected on contemporary populations and sometimes to data reconstructed for historical populations. Reviewing the various components, we find that:

1. Estimates of *fecundability* have come from varied contexts, modern as well as historical (although, for the former, it is not always easy to go

1. With some exceptions like Anabaptist sects of North America.

from "residual" fecundability, that is, including some practice of contraception, to "natural" fecundability).

2. Our ideas on *intrauterine mortality* are solely the result of recent observations; since there is no solidly based opinion on the degree of variation in time or space of the rate of intrauterine mortality, we are obliged to accept for the past the results obtained for the present.

3. The duration of the *postpartum nonsusceptible period* is very dependent on the duration and the frequency of breast-feeding, which have diminished considerably; this dependence has been measured (at least indirectly) for historical as well as modern populations, and the results in the two cases are consistent.

4. The incidence of *sterility*, and its increase with age, are almost impossible to measure in populations which practice contraception (even to a limited extent); lacking recent estimates, we must be satisfied with accepting those established for historical populations.

Role Played by Nuptiality

In determining the level of fertility, the marital customs prevalent in society play an important role. Although these are primarily *social* variables and thus do not enter directly into our analysis, they are not "birth control" variables. One can see, in the types of union, age at marriage, conditions or obligations of remarriage after widowhood, consequences of marital infidelity, and so forth, not only society's view of *reproduction*, the conditions and limits of this essential function, but also a good deal of its attitude toward *social organization*, the relations between individuals, functions devolved to the family, and so on. The important point here is that the level of fertility is greatly affected by these practices, since the final number of children a woman has depends *first* on the number of years that she has lived "in unions," and on the nature of these unions.

For example, in a study of the birth cohorts of 1914–28 in Martinique (Leridon 1971, ref. 348),[2] the relatively low level of fertility could be explained by the following reasons:

1. The fertility specific to unions other than marriages (common law and visiting) was about 18% less than that within marriages; as a result, fertility was 7% lower than if all the unions had been of the "marriage" type alone.

2. The interruptions between successive unions led to an additional reduction of 10%; in the group 25–29 years, for example, only 70% of all years lived were spent in unions, although 72% of the women had already entered into a union at age 25, and 88% at age 30.

2. Some of the results of this article (on page 284) are incorrect due to an error which did not affect the rest of the article; the correct figures are given here.

3. A higher incidence of sterility in the cohorts involved could be responsible for a reduction in fertility of about 7% in comparison with a situation of "normal" sterility.

Finally, a woman married at age 20 and remaining in a union until age 50 would have had 7.9 children on the average (8.5 if sterility had been lower); this was reduced to 6.4 children because some marriages started later than age 20 or were dissolved before age 50; to 6.0 children owing to the existence of unions other than marriage, with lower fertility; and to 5.4 by the interruptions between unions.

Of course, it is possible to eliminate the effect of nuptiality by considering only the fertility of married women (in the widest sense of the term, i.e., of all women involved in a type of union recognized as normal by the society in question); but the final level of fertility will depend on the structure of nuptiality, and it is interesting to measure this effect.

Age-Specific Fertility Rates: Completed Fertility

Table 7.1 shows observations from historical or contemporary populations. Besides the *age-specific legitimate fertility rates*, there are also:

1. *mean number of children by completed family*, for a woman married at age 20—mean number of children per woman entering into a union at age 20 and surviving in it until at least 45 (without widowhood or divorce); this number is obtained by multiplying by 0.005 the sum of the legitimate fertility rates for age groups 20–24 and above; and
2. *completed fertility*—the mean number of children per woman surviving to 45 years (including the effects of celibacy, widowhood, and divorce); this figure was not always given in the studies in question and has not been possible to estimate in all cases (most often owing to the lack of data on widowhood).

Comparing these two indexes, we find that the difference between the two figures is small where the amount of celibacy is small, the age at marriage very low, and mortality low (and the risk of widowhood thus reduced). For example, among the Hutterites and the Amish it is between 10% and 15%. If, on the contrary, many women remain single, if the mean age at marriage is clearly well over 20 years, and if the risk of widowhood is high (and remarriage not immediate), the difference between the two figures may reach 50%. Such is the case with historical France, where a woman reaching 45 years of age and married at least once had an average of 4 to 6 children, while the average completed family size for a woman who married at 20 years and remained in union until 45 years of age often exceeded 8 children.

In some cases the mean number of children per woman surviving to 45 years can exceed the fertility of completed families (cf. the case of Senegal).

Table 7.1. Fertility in Selected Noncontracepting Populations

Population	Ref.	Marital Fertility Rates (per 1,000)						Mean Number of Children	
		15–19 years	20–24 years	25–29 years	30–34 years	35–39 years	40–44 years	45–49 years	Completed Families, Women Married at Age 20 (1)	All Women Surviving to Age 50 (2)
Non-European populations										
Bengal Hindu villages (marriages 1945–46)	350	118	323	288	282	212	100	33	6.2	—
Punjab Chamars villages (women born 1900–1914)	352	277	370	357	346	259	113	—	7.2	—
Senegal (Siné-Saloun) (births 1963–65)	322	280	340	306	260	182	92	28	6.1[c]	6.7
Martinique (women born 1914–28)	348	621	481	440	333	211	114	11	7.9	5.4
Villages near Bombay[e] (births 1954–55)	325	194	286	289	241	156	84	28	5.4	5.3
Average (5 series)		298	360	336	292	204	101	25	6.6	—
Populations originating from Europe										
Canada (marriages 1700–1730)	335	493	509	495	484	410	231	30	10.8	8.0[b]
Hutterites (USA) (marriages 1921–30)	328	—	550	502	447	406	222	61	10.9	9.5[b]
Amish (USA) (women born 1900–1920)	324	83	365	462	251	221	82	14	7.0	6.33[a]

(Continued on page 108)

Table 7.1.—Continued

Population	Ref.	Marital Fertility Rates (per 1,000)							Mean Number of Children	
		15–19 years	20–24 years	25–29 years	30–34 years	35–39 years	40–44 years	45–49 years	Completed Families, Women Married at Age 20 (1)	All Women Surviving to Age 50 (2)
European populations										
Geneva (bourgeoisie) (husbands born before 1600)	336	264	389	362	327	275	123	19	7.5	—
Geneva (bourgeoisie) (husbands born 1600–1649)	336	419	525	485	429	287	141	16	9.4	—
Norway (years 1871–75)	339	433	426	393	332	281	166	40	8.2	—
Sweden (marriages 1841–1900)	345	—	319	332	279	226	122	12	6.4	—
Anhausen (Germany) (marriages 1692–1799)	346	—	472	496	450	355	173	37	9.9	—
Colyton (England) (marriages 1560–1629)	360	412	467	403	369	302	174	18	8.7	—
France: Northwest (marriages 1670–1769)	341	317	447	426	380	293	150	10	8.5	—
France: Southwest (marriages 1720–69)	337	275	404	363	343	260	146	22	7.7	—
Average (8 series)		353	431	407	364	285	149	22	8.3	—

French villages

Boulay (Moselle) (marriages before 1780)	343	433	480	452	391	341	183	27	9.4	—
Bilhères d'Ossau (Béarn) (marriages 1740–79)	329	198	414	400	353	319	165	13	8.3	—
Crulai (Normandy) (marriages 1674–1742)	332	324	428	431	359	319	119	10	8.3	5.6[b]
Ile-de-France (marriages 1740–79)	331	461	527	515	448	368	144	21	10.1	6.1[b]
Sotteville (Normandy) (marriages 1760–90)[d]	333	—	491	440	429	297	125	10	9.0	—
Thézels Saint-Sernin (Quercy) (marriages 1700–1791)	358	208	385	335	290	242	67	0	6.6	3.7[b]
Tourouvre (Perche) (marriages 1665–1714)	323	236	412	425	378	330	164	11	8.6	6.0[b]
Average (7 series)		310	448	428	378	317	138	12	8.6	
Average series										
13 series from various countries (Henry)	340	—	435	407	371	298	152	22	8.4	—
38 series from villages in France and Germany (Smith)	354	—	475	450	398	316	158	—	9.0	—

(1) Sum of the marital fertility rates after 20 (÷1,000).
(2) Sum of general fertility rates (÷1,000).
[a] Ever-married women.
[b] Estimated by the present author.
[c] Marital fertility rates were estimated from general fertility rates by dividing the latter by the proportion of ever-married women in the same group.
[d] Families with prenuptial conceptions excluded.
[e] Fertility in the four villages where the decline had not started. Adapted from the discussion of the original data by L. Henry (*Population* 15[1960]: 144–47).

This is true when fertility and proportion of women married are high before age 20, for this part of reproductive life is not taken into account in our definition of "completed families."

Finally, taking into account the proportion of women who remain single and those who die before reaching age 45, the *net reproduction rate* in populations where mortality is fairly high is generally reduced to little above 1. For example, in the study on Crulai the mean expectancy of life at birth for women was about 30 years; according to the United Nations life tables, the proportion of women surviving up to age 30 would be 0.470 in such a case. It follows a net reproduction rate close to $R_0 = 0.488 \times 0.470 \times 5.6 = 1.28$.

When considering only the fertility of married women, the most striking fact of table 7.1 is the wide dispersion of results: the size of completed families may actually vary by 100%, and the same is true for each age-specific rate.

Besides these considerable differences of levels, we may also note that the schedules are not all similar: for example, the ratio of the rate for 35–39 years to the rate for 25–29 years ranges from 0.48 (Amish, Martinique) to 0.83 (Canada) or 0.81 (Hutterites). This is due to the specific influence of the various components: fecundability and the nonsusceptible period determine mostly the *overall level* of the rates, while the progression of sterility with age determines the *evolution of the rates with age*. This could also be due to some kind of birth control practice, increasing with the number of children already born.

Among more homogeneous subgroups, however, such as the seven French towns or villages, the profiles are more similar to each other (the ratio cited above ranging only from 0.67 to 0.80), although total fertility is still quite variable (6.6 to 10.1 live births).

Birth Intervals

The mean duration of successive birth intervals is obviously related to the fertility rate: the longer the interval, the lower the fertility. The relation between these two measures of the same phenomenon is, however, far from simple.

It is true that the mean interval tends to equal the inverse of the fertility rate (after some years of marriage) under the following conditions: fecundability, nonsusceptible period, and intrauterine mortality homogeneous and constant; no sterility. This result has especially been established by Henry (cf. chap. 9). In reality, these conditions are evidently not fulfilled. However, if we consider only the fertility of women who are later fertile (i.e., excluding the effects of sterility), and if the heterogeneity of the other variables is not too great, the relationship is still approximately verified for births occurring between 20 and 35 years of age. For all women (fertile later or not), the fertility rate will be slightly less than the inverse of the interval between births (the difference being about 10% between 25 and 35 years of age).

Thus the interpretation of differences between mean intervals observed in two populations must be done with caution. Let us take the example of a group of "completed" families, that is, families where the women are at least 45 years old and the unions were not broken by widowhood or divorce before that age. According to the data of table 7.1, we would expect the successive

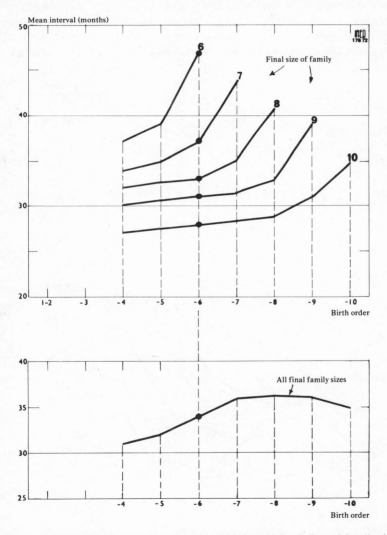

Fig. 7.1. Birth intervals: Study by order of birth and final size of family (data adjusted from Okasaki 1951, ref. 351).

intervals between births, rank by rank, to increase regularly, since the fertility rates decrease regularly as the woman moves further along in her reproductive period; this should be especially true at the end of the reproductive period, when fertility rates are very low. Actually, however, the successive intervals tend to reach a plateau and even to decrease for higher ranks.

The paradox is resolved if the mean birth interval is recomputed for *each completed family size*. A very clear lengthening of the last one or two intervals is then observed, no matter what the size of the family at completed fertility. With this second method of computation the number of observations is equal for all the birth ranks within each series. With the first method, on the other hand, the weighting is not uniform, since there is no interval of a higher

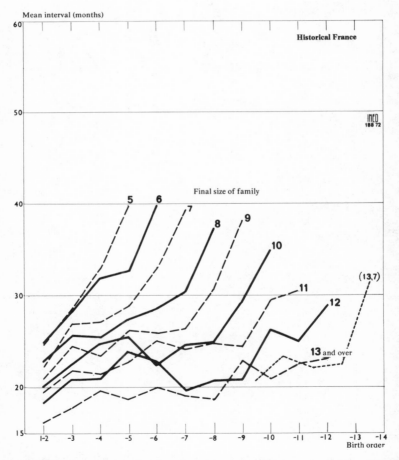

Fig. 7.2. Birth intervals, by order and final size of family (historical France).

rank than *n* in the families whose size is smaller than or equal to *n*. Figure 7.1 illustrates this point.

The advantage to grouping intervals by final family size lies in the possibility of then comparing successive intervals. The variations observed can be related to the *progression of the rank or of the mother's age*, and it is not easy to dissociate the two. As far as we know, the most important variable for biological factors is age, as the previous chapters have shown.

Data on birth intervals classified by rank and final family size are very few. Because of random variations, it is necessary to have a fairly large number of completed families (several hundred). Only two examples will be given here: one a group of families of historical France (eighteenth century), reconstructed from data of several studies in historical demography (Leridon 1967, ref. 029),

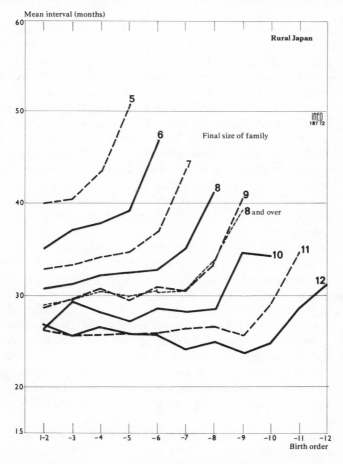

Fig. 7.3.   Birth intervals, by order and final size of family (rural Japan).

and the other a group of rural families in Japan, surveyed in 1940 by Okasaki (1951, ref. 351). Only completed families of at least five children have been considered here; these numbered 450 in the first sample and 3,000 in the second. (See Appendix tables B1 and B2 for data.)

Figures 7.2 and 7.3 show the same pattern as figure 7.1: a very clear increase in the last interval (about 6 to 7 months), whatever the final family size; a more moderate increase in the next-to-last interval; and a tiering of the curves by final family size. Since permanent sterility plays no part in these results (by definition, each woman is still fecund at the time of her last conception), the lengthening of intervals can be explained only by the evolution of the other components (fecundability, intrauterine mortality, nonsusceptible period). I have tried to take advantage of the characteristics of these networks in order to study the possible evolution of fecundability with age, in an analysis which is developed in Appendix A.

Before completing the brief examination of these networks, let us check the relationship between birth intervals and fertility rates mentioned above. In the region from which the historical French sample was taken, women married at 25 years of age on the average. Final family size for completed families was, on the average, between 6 and 7 children. Taking the mean of the intervals between births 2 and 3, and between births 3 and 4, in families of 6 and 7 children (cf. Appendix table B2), we obtain 28.6 months, which would correspond to an annual fertility rate of 0.420. Taking account of the mean age at marriage and the mean size of the first three birth intervals, this rate would apply to the group 30–34 years. Table 7.1 shows the means calculated for the seven series from French villages (half of which are also our interval sample). The rate for 30–34 years is 0.378, or 10% below the value obtained from the birth intervals. The difference is consistent with the deviation mentioned above.

Finally, it should be repeated that there is always difficulty in obtaining estimates of fertility, especially in following its evolution over time, from birth intervals. As we have seen, there are two major problems:

1. *The truncation effect*, whose various manifestations have been analyzed at length in the articles by Henry (1953, ref. 285; 1961, ref. 283) and by Sheps et al. (1970, ref. 034, 1973 ref. 313). To characterize this effect, let us merely say that the process of reproduction cannot be considered as stationary, homogeneous, and of "infinite" duration. Whether the investigation is terminated at a given point in time (as in the case of a sample survey) or at a given age (even if one continues to 45 or 50 years of age, i.e., to the end of the reproductive period), the length of observation is always limited. This introduces various selection biases.

2. The importance of weighting resulting from the sampling method or the method of computation (see Wolfers 1968, ref. 039 or Sheps and Menken 1972, ref. 035).

Let me quote in conclusion the last lines of the article by Sheps et al. (1970 ref. 034):

> It is clear that despite the arguments in favor of birth interval analysis, the difficulties of interpreting such analyses are great. Considerably more exploration is needed before we can be certain of the usefulness or interpretation of survey data on closed or open birth intervals.
> It is doubtful whether the current emphasis on data for such intervals as an index of changing natality patterns is justified.

Estimates through a Simulation Model

I shall now relate the results obtained at a macrodemographic level, that is, in terms of fertility rates or mean number of children, to those given in the preceding chapters on a microdemographic level, that is, relative to each component. It is very rare to have available *for the same population* estimates for all the components at once. It is necessary, therefore, to make use of a model into which we can enter simultaneously the information actually available and reasonable estimates for the unknown variables. Since chapter 9 is devoted entirely to the presentation and discussion of various types of possible models, only a brief description will be given here.

The model used here is a simulation based on the "Monte Carlo" method which allows great flexibility even with complex hypotheses. The model, called SIMNAT, is a version, with no contraception, of the SIMULA model described in chapter 9. The various components are treated in the following way:[3]

1. *Permanent sterility* occurs at an age S_x which is defined for each woman at the beginning of the process (at 15 years of age), from a distribution which is part of the input.
2. *Fecundability* varies from one woman to another, and also varies with age and as a function of age at permanent sterility. The maximum value for the fecundability of each woman (FMAX) is defined by random drawing from an approximately normal distribution. From 15 to 20 years of age, fecundability increases linearly from an initial value (FPUB = 0.10) to FMAX; from 20 years to an age equal to $(S_x - 12.5)$, it is equal to FMAX; and from $(S_x - 12.5)$ to S_x, it decreases linearly until it reaches zero. If $(S_x - 12.5)$ is smaller than 20, the linear decrement takes place between the ages of 20 and S_x: the rate of decline is thus dependent on the age at onset of permanent sterility. Finally, if S_x is lower than 20, sterility simply interrupts the age-dependent increase in fecundability.

---

3. See Appendix tables B4 to B7 for detailed data. The choice of hypotheses is justified in chapter 9.

The reason for this rather complex procedure is the following. In Appendix A, I show (through a deterministic model) that the specific increase in last intervals of all families is due to a decrease of effective fecundability before the age at onset of permanent sterility, *whatever this age* (at least after 30 or 35 years). Fecundability is thus dependent both on current age and on age at sterility.

3. *Intrauterine mortality* increases with age at the tempo indicated in chapter 4, for a mean rate of 15% (cf. p. 64); the risk is identical for all women of the same age.

4. *The duration of the nonsusceptible period* is determined at the moment of each conception; two distributions are used, according to whether the pregnancy results in a live birth or an intrauterine death.

5. Each woman begins her exposure to the risk of conception only at *marriage*; a series of monthly probabilities of marriage is used. This model does not take into account divorce, widowhood, or risk of death for the woman, although infant mortality is taken into account through the distribution of the duration of the nonsusceptible period. Thus we obtain the fertility of completed families, either for a given age at marriage or for a given distribution of ages at marriage. The size of each cohort (one set of hypotheses) is 1,000.

The intention here is to measure the relative importance of each component in determining the level of fertility. The basic theoretical situation is one in which all women marry at age 15 (and remain in the union until age 45), become sterile only after age 45, and do not breast-feed their children. Under these conditions, the mean nonsusceptible period for a live birth is 11.7 months (including gestation); the risk of intrauterine mortality is about 12% from 20 to 25 years, and reaches 32% at 45 years; and mean fecundability at 20–25 years is fixed at 0.25.

These hypotheses do attempt to be realistic. Although there is no population where all women marry at age 15 and remain fecund until age 45, this may be the case for at least *some* women. Under these conditions, each woman would have, on the average, 17.5 children; this figure is the basis of tables 7.2 and 7.3.

The effect of sterility is now considered. The "low sterility" hypothesis corresponds to estimates proposed by Henry and Vincent for European populations (cf. chap. 6). Here, the mean age of onset of sterility is 41 years. This probably is not an absolute minimum, but rather applies to a population subject to fairly good socioeconomic conditions. If the other hypotheses are unchanged, each woman would have 15.3 children (or 87% of the figure given above).

It is not an easy matter to propose higher estimates for the risk of sterility. The "high" estimate was defined first by assuming the same rates of sterility to be reached five years earlier than in the "low" estimate. The reason for this

Table 7.2. Levels of Natural Fertility (Estimated through a Simulation Model)

Sterility (1)	Nonsusceptible Period (N.S.P.) (2)	Marriage at the Age of 15	Early Marriage (3)	Late Marriage (3)
Low sterility	No breast-feeding	15.2	12.8	8.1
	Short N.S.P.	12.3	10.3	6.5
	Long N.S.P.	10.0	8.4	5.3
Median sterility	No breast-feeding	13.5	11.4	7.2
	Short N.S.P.	10.8	9.1	5.8
	Long N.S.P.	8.7	7.4	4.7
High sterility	No breast-feeding	12.1	10.2	6.5
	Short N.S.P.	9.6	8.1	5.1
	Long N.S.P.	7.9	6.7	4.2

Low fecundability—the above values were computed with a mean fecundability equal to 0.25 at the age of 20–25; if fecundability has *half* the assumed value, they must be multiplied by a coefficient ranging from 0.75 (no breast-feeding, late marriage) to 0.83 (long N.S.P., early marriage).

NOTE: This table gives the number of live births per woman that would occur under the stated assumptions. A woman being fecund and married from the age of 15 to 45, not breast-feeding her children, would have on the average 17.5 children (in the absence of mortality).
(1) Low sterility: proportions of permanently sterile couples by age estimated by Henry (mean age at onset of sterility = 41 years).
High sterility: Same proportions applied to couples 5 years younger (mean age = 36 years).
(2) Nonsusceptible period (including duration of pregnancy):
Long: average = 22 months (24 for a child surviving up to 1 year; corresponds to a duration of breast-feeding close to 24 months).
Short: average = 16 months.
(3) Early marriage = Asiatic and African type (mean = 19 years; no celibacy).
Late marriage = European type, eighteenth century (mean = 25 years; celibacy = 8%).

choice is that, as we have seen (chap. 1), in a population like India's women could reach menopause 5 years earlier, on the average, than in European populations. This hypothesis, however, involves a reduction in fertility rates after age 35 which is too rapid and thus is probably excessive. A "medium" hypothesis has thus been established by assuming that the 5-year difference exists only up to age 25 and decreases progressively thereafter so as to be only two years at the end of the reproductive career. Under this hypothesis, the mean number of children is 13.5, or 77% of the initial figure.

Next, breast-feeding is introduced, in order to define a new distribution of the nonsusceptible period (corresponding to a live birth). The "long non-susceptible period" hypothesis represents a situation of widespread breast-feeding, over about 24 months. If the child survives to 1 year of age, the duration of postpartum sterility is, on the average, 15.3 months. If the child dies

Table 7.3. Range of Variation in Natural Fertility (Estimated through a Simulation Model)

Sterility (1)	Nonsusceptible Period (N.S.P.) (2)	Marriage at the Age of 15	Early Marriage (3)	Late Marriage (3)
Low sterility	No breast-feeding	0.87	0.73	0.46
	Short N.S.P.	0.70	0.59	0.37
	Long N.S.P.	0.57	0.48	0.30
Medium sterility	No breast-feeding	0.77	0.65	0.41
	Short N.S.P.	0.62	0.52	0.33
	Long N.S.P.	0.50	0.42	0.27
High sterility	No breast-feeding	0.69	0.58	0.37
	Short N.S.P.	0.55	0.46	0.29
	Long N.S.P.	0.45	0.38	0.24

Low fecundability—the above values were computed with a mean fecundability equal to 0.25 at the age of 20–25; if fecundability has *half* the assumed value, they must be multiplied by a coefficient ranging from 0.75 (no breast-feeding, late marriage) to 0.83 (long N.S.P., early marriage).

NOTE: This table gives the number of live births that would occur under the stated assumptions, for one birth that would have occurred to a woman fecund and married from the age of 15 to 45, not breast-feeding her children (such a woman would have 17.5 children on the average, in the absence of mortality).
(1) Low sterility: proportions of permanently sterile couples by age estimated by Henry (mean age at onset of sterility = 41 years).
High sterility: Same proportions applied to couples 5 years younger (mean age = 36 years).
(2) Nonsusceptible period (including duration of pregnancy):
Long: average = 22 months (24 for a child surviving up to 1 year; corresponds to a duration of breast-feeding close to 24 months).
Short: average = 16 months.
(3) Early marriage = Asiatic and African type (mean = 19 years; no celibacy).
Late marriage = European type, eighteenth century (mean = 25 years; celibacy = 8%).

before 1 year, amenorrhea is assumed to cease immediately. The preceding distribution has thus been combined with the distribution of deaths during the first 12 months, for an infant mortality rate of about 200 per 1,000. Finally, the mean duration of the nonsusceptible period is 21.8 months (including 9 months of gestation).

The "short nonsusceptible period" hypothesis is obtained by combining a distribution of long nonsusceptible periods with a distribution of nonsusceptible periods with no breast-feeding (weighting each 50%). The overall mean is 15.8 months. This corresponds either to a situation where breast-feeding occurs but is not widespread or to a situation where breast-feeding is widespread but shorter (by about 9 months).

Finally, the distributions of age at marriage are taken into account. In the "early marriage" hypothesis, the mean age is 19 years and permanent celibacy is negligible, which corresponds to nuptiality of the Asiatic or African type. The "late marriage" hypothesis leaves 8% of the women never married at 45 years; for the others, mean age at marriage is 25 years. This distribution represents the situation of northwest France in the eighteenth century.

Let us now return to tables 7.2 and 7.3. Table 7.2 shows the mean number of children born to a woman who survives to 50 years of age and whose union (if she was ever married) was never broken. Table 7.3 shows the same numbers, expressed as a proportion of *one* birth that would have occurred under the basic hypothesis (continuous fecundity from 15 to 45 years of age). The outlined section is considered the most realistic: most real situations should in principle be located there (by interpolation between model situations if necessary).

The range of variation is considerable. Even when considering only the outlined section of the table, the mean number of children falls from 12.8 (early marriage, no breast-feeding, low sterility) to 4.7 (late marriage, long breast-feeding, medium sterility). The ratio of these two numbers is 2.7:1.

The case of the Hutterites (9.5 children per married woman) could be represented by a combination of hypotheses such as low sterility, short breast-feeding, and marriage somewhat later than the "early marriage" hypothesis (they married on the average at 20.7 years, or 2 years later than in the given hypothesis). The population of Crulai, with 6.2 children per woman, corresponds to the combination late marriage, low sterility, short or medium breast-feeding. It is important to remember, in comparing tables 7.1 and 7.2, that the last column of table 7.1 represents the mean number of children for women surviving to 50 years, *including those whose union was dissolved by widowhood or divorce*, while the results of table 7.2 do not take these factors into account (though they could be included in the assumptions on sterility, since the effect of the loss of spouse is equivalent to a sterilization).

On the whole, I believe these results are more useful in measuring the relative influence of each component than in trying to situate any specific conditions. This is the point of view adopted in table 7.3, where only relative numbers are given.

The effect of fecundability has also been examined by making several runs with a mean fecundability reduced by half. Fertility decreased by only 17% to 25%, according to whether the periods of exposure to risk were greater or lesser relative to the periods of nonexposure (celibacy and nonsusceptible period).

In summary, this study by means of a model confirms two things: (1) the range of situations of "uncontrolled" fertility (fertility in the absence of contraception) is wide; and (2) the same level of fertility may be reached with various combinations of values of each component.

Natural Fertility and Contraception

To conclude both this chapter and the analysis of the several components of fertility, we can now define "conditions of natural fertility" as any situation in which there is no conscious attempt on the part of individuals or of couples to limit the number of births. With this definition, all behavior that does not explicitly intend to decrease fertility would not alter the "natural" aspect of fertility conditions.

It is therefore evident that collective behavior and individual behavior do have a part in natural fertility, as well as physiological variables. Matrimonial customs, frequency of sexual intercourse, periods of separation of spouses, frequency and duration of lactation, and so forth, contribute to the fertility level of each population.

Even assuming these variables to be identical for two populations, their fertility could still differ considerably owing to differences in nutritional and sanitary conditions: frequency of anovular cycles, intrauterine mortality, duration of postpartum amenorrhea, age of onset of permanent sterility, and so forth, probably depend on the quantity and quality of food and the level of sanitation.

It is only after "controlling" for this group of variables that one can turn to *genetic* differences between populations or, in other terms, can define the "intrinsic" fertility of a population. In actual fact, this would be largely a theoretical exercise, since fertility has been shown to be only the *result* of a whole series of behavioral factors that are themselves greatly influenced by social constraints.

What still remains to be considered, of course, is behavior that aims to control the number or spacing of births for an individual—that is, contraception. Chapter 8 and part of chapter 9 will be devoted to this, in order to show that the microdemographic approach used in most of the preceding chapters is also perfectly suited to taking this new dimension into account.

8

Contraception, Abortion, and Sterilization

How Is Each Component Affected?

There are simple ways to include the various means of limiting births into the present framework. The practice of *contraception* induces a decrease in the monthly risk of conception; thus, instead of its "natural" value, fecundability will have a lower, *residual* value that is a function of the effectiveness of the contraceptive method used. The practice of induced abortion may be taken into account by modifying the risk of intrauterine mortality; abortion is generally performed during the third month of pregnancy, a duration close to the mean length of gestation in cases of recognizable spontaneous abortions. Finally, voluntary sterilization ends the reproductive period, usually in an irreversible way, just as naturally acquired sterility would do.

However, these new variables can no longer be analyzed principally as functions of the woman's age; rather, they depend on the duration of marriage and, more precisely, on the number of children already born. That is, what will modify contraceptive effectiveness, frequency of recourse to induced abortion, or motivation for voluntary sterilization is each woman's (or each couple's) previous fertile experience. Thus, in developing the models as well as in analyzing each component, the pertinent variable will usually be the number of children already born rather than the woman's age.

Effectiveness of Contraception: Theory

Since the first works of R. Pearl in the 1930s, the notion of the effectiveness of a contraceptive method has been made more and more precise, notably thanks to R. G. Potter and C. Tietze; but there is still some distance between theoretical refinements and practical usages.

In the theoretical area, the situation has been clarified by distinguishing three levels in measuring the effectiveness of contraception:

1. *theoretical* or *physiological effectiveness*, measured under the ideal conditions of use of the method without negligence, by subjects acting under "laboratory" (-type) conditions;

2. *use-effectiveness*, which corresponds to normal use in a real population, where people are not all well motivated or educated;

3. *extended use-effectiveness*, in which the cases of discontinuation of the method are taken into account; here, a pregnancy following discontinuation of a method, for example, when the method is not well tolerated, is also considered to be a failure of the method.

Much of the confusion in the debate over the use of contraceptive methods results from the mixing of these various levels. As we shall see in the next section, the classification of various methods differs greatly according to whether their theoretical effectiveness or their use-effectiveness is considered. Likewise, the acceptability and continuation rate of a method must be considered important elements in evaluating its "effectiveness" in the broad sense. This will be especially true for the question of "demographic effectiveness" of a method—that is, the effect of its use on general indexes of fertility.

For the moment, let us remain on the individual level. Strictly speaking, effectiveness (theoretical or in use) is measured by the reduction of the risk of fertilization it entails. If $P(\text{Nat.})$ is "natural" fecundability in the absence of contraception and $P(\text{Res.})$ is "residual" fecundability with contraception, the effectiveness (E) of a method can be defined as follows: $E = 1 - P(\text{Res.})/P(\text{Nat.})$.

The link with our framework is thus established. Unfortunately, this concept allows us to measure effectiveness (E) only if we know both $P(\text{Nat.})$ and $P(\text{Res.})$; but these can be measured only in particular situations (such as at the beginning of marriage) that are not our primary interest here. We must thus introduce a much more practical index, developed by R. Pearl (1938, ref. 083).

The simplest method of measuring contraceptive effectiveness might be to determine by a survey the total number of pregnancies recorded among a group of women and the number of pregnancies that were "unwanted" by these women; the ratio of the latter to the former would give the proportion of pregnancies that were unwanted, a figure which could be considered an index of the ineffectiveness of contraception. In fact, however, this figure is rather ambiguous for several reasons.

First of all, it does not take the time factor into account: it would probably be higher for the first 10 years of marriage than for the first 5 years; there are thus problems in comparing results from different sources.

Second, the lack of precision about whether a pregnancy was "wanted" or "unwanted" may be great; in particular, there is a clear tendency to rationalize a posteriori the size of the completed family, even if it does not correspond to initial aspirations.

Finally, there is a risk of attributing to contraception some successes that result from the onset of sterility in a couple.

The index proposed by R. Pearl removes the second objection completely and the two others partially. In a cohort of women (e.g., newly married), one calculates the ratio:

$$R = \frac{\text{total number of pregnancies recorded}}{\text{number of months of exposure to risk}} \times 1{,}200,$$

which is called "number of pregnancies per 100 woman-years."

In calculating the numerator, all pregnancies are counted, whether wanted or not. For the denominator one excludes periods of separation, pregnancy, amenorrhea, and sterility.

One disadvantage is that this index still depends on the length of the period of observation, owing to the heterogeneity of the group (with respect to natural fecundability and individual effectiveness of contraception). There is a selection effect, since women with a high residual fecundability conceive in a shorter time on the average, and thus are the first to be excluded; the apparent pregnancy rate becomes lower over time, as can be seen in table 8.1, resulting from an American survey.

One way of surmounting this problem is to standardize the length of the observation period—for example, at 12 months. But in practice the temptation of including in the data either shorter or longer periods is rarely resisted.

It should be noted that this index cannot be interpreted as the "number of births observed in a population" in one year. Actually, only the periods of exposure to risk are taken into account; we are counting *ovulations*, not months lived. When expressed per 100 woman-years, the index could reach

Table 8.1.   Effect of Length of Observation Period on Pearl Index

Length of Observation Period	R (per 100 woman years)
1 month	42.4
≤6 months	37.1
≤12 months	35.7
≤18 months	30.8
≤24 months	29.4
≤36 months	27.3
≤48 months	26.2

SOURCES: Westoff, Potter, Sagi, Mishler: *Family Growth in Metropolitan America* (Princeton: Princeton University Press, 1961).

a value of 1,200 if all women conceived each time they were exposed to the risk of conception (i.e., if natural fecundability equaled 1). In practice, with fecundability of around 0.2, the index would be about 300 per 100 woman-years, while the corresponding usual fertility rate in the population would be between 30 and 60 per 100 (depending on whether the women were breast-feeding their children). This must be kept in mind when comparing situations with and without contraception.

It is not easy to relate the Pearl index (R) to effectiveness (E), except for values of R limited to the first month (R_1); in this latter case: $R_1 = 1,200\ P(\text{Nat.})(1 - E)$.

Henry has proposed (1968, ref. 412) some approximate relations between values of R_{12} (calculated for 12 months) and of E, as shown in table 8.2.

Table 8.2. Relation between the Pearl Index (R_{12}) and Effectiveness of Contraception (E)

R_{12}	E (%)
1.5 to 2	99.5
3 to 4	99
6 to 8	98
12 to 21	95
About 30	90

SOURCE: Henry 1968 (ref. 412).

Discontinuations and failures of a contraceptive method can be analyzed simultaneously using the multiple decrement life table method. The methodology, which has been set forth by Potter (1967, ref. 418; see also Freedman and Takeshita 1969, ref. 364b: Appendix X-2), is quite similar to the one described in chapter 4 for intrauterine mortality. Let us take, for example, the case of the insertion of an IUD. The end of the period of use of the contraceptive could be a result of the expulsion of the IUD, or of its voluntary withdrawal, or of a conception. From a followup survey of a group of women, then, it is possible to calculate month by month how many are still protected by their IUD, also taking into account those lost from observation. Let:

E_x be the number of devices expelled during month x,

R_x be the number of devices removed during month x,

P_x be the number of new pregnancies during month x,

N_x be the number of women still protected at the beginning of month x, and

W_x be the number of withdrawals from observation during month x.

These withdrawals are of two types: the stopping of observation, decided by the observer, or the withdrawal from observation, decided by the woman. In the second case there could be some correlation between the withdrawal and the other events, creating a bias in the analysis: the risk of a pregnancy during month x, for example, could be different for women still under observation at month x and for those lost before month x.

For each type of outcome, specific rates (also called "net rates" by Tietze) can be calculated: the conditional probabilities of an expulsion, a removal, or a pregnancy during month x, for a woman who retains the device at time x, are respectively:

$$Q_{xe} = E_x/(N_x - 0.5W_x),$$
$$Q_{xr} = R_x/(N_x - 0.5W_x),$$
$$Q_{xp} = P_x/(N_x - 0.5W_x).$$

These rates are *additive* within any one month, and it is thus easy to compute overall rates of discontinuation and of continuation.

Inversely, if we want to study a simple risk as if it were the only one operating in the population, we would construct a single decrement life table, specific of this risk. For instance, the conditional probability of expelling the device during month x, in the absence of competing events, would be

$$q_{xe} = \frac{E_x}{N_x - 0.5(P_x + R_x + W_x)}.$$

In this case, the rates coming from different life tables are *not* additive, but the number of events derived from the tables *are* additive.

Effectiveness of Contraception: Results

The wide variation in failure rates *for any one method*, found when compiling results from different studies, is striking. We are dealing here, of course, with the use-effectiveness of the contraceptive, and, as mentioned previously, this depends mostly on the degree of motivation and the level of education of the couples involved. Under the best of circumstances, the use-effectiveness of a method can approach its theoretical effectiveness. For example, the temperature method, if strictly practiced by women who know how to interpret their temperature curves and who abstain from intercourse during the required periods, may be as effective as hormonal contraception. On the other hand, the same method practiced in a lax way would produce a failure rate 30 to 50 times as high.

Also, there is widespread confusion in the calculation of failure rates. They are calculated sometimes as simply the number of pregnancies recorded in one year per 100 "acceptors"; sometimes as Pearl's index; or sometimes by a life table method, yielding either *net* rates (competing events) or *crude* rates (a single event). The longer the period considered, and the higher the various rates, the wider the discrepancies that result.

Table 8.3. Failure Rates and Continuation Rates for Various Contraceptive Methods and Sterilization

Method	Failure Rates[a] Theoretical	Clinical	Use-effectiveness (E) %	Continuation Rates (%) 1 Year	2 Years
Tubal sterilization	0.04–0.08	0.04–0.08	~100		
Vasectomy	0.15	0.15–1.0	99.9		
Injection	?	0.3–2.5	99.5–99.9	40–85	25–80
Oral contraceptives					
Combined	0.03–0.10⎫				
Sequential	0.20–0.56⎬ 1–7		98–99.5	40–80	30–70
Minipill	1.6 –3.0⎭				
Temperature					
rhythm	0.07–1.3	1–25	90–99.5		
IUD	1.0–3.0	1–10	98–99.5	50–85	40–75
Diaphragm	1.5–3.0	3–35	90–99		
Condom	1.5–3.0	3–35	90–99		
Vaginal (chemical)	(1.8)	2–40	50–99		
Calendar rhythm	(3.8)	15–50	50–95		
Coitus					
interruptus	(3–10)	(10–100)	–		
No contraception	–	150–300	0		

SOURCES: Most theoretical rates are taken from Tietze 1971 (ref. 426); most clinical rates and continuation rates are taken from various issues of *Population Reports*, 1973–75.
[a] Number of pregnancies per 100 couple-years of exposure; whenever possible, the rate was computed for the *first 12 months* of exposure.

For these two reasons, table 8.3 shows *ranges* of effectiveness, sometimes fairly wide, within which fall most estimates for the method considered. The first column gives the theoretical failure rates, and the methods are ranked in decreasing order of effectiveness; the second column gives the clinical failure rates. For some methods (the modern ones, used in well-educated populations) the observed failure rates are usually close to the lower limit, while for others (the traditional ones) these observed rates are close to the upper limit. Another distinction may be made between contraception for spacing and contraception for ending births: in the former case the motivation will be weak and failures fairly frequent; in the latter case motivation will be strong, and even methods usually regarded as undependable can be surprisingly effective. This was a notable result of the "Family Growth in Metropolitan America" survey (see, for example, C. Westoff, R. G. Potter, and P. C. Sagi: *The Third Child* [Princeton: Princeton University Press, 1963]).

The third column gives an approximate relationship between the clinical failure rate and use-effectiveness, as proposed by Henry. We must not be fooled by the high values of effectiveness: although a method which is "50% effective" may have some considerable effect on the reproduction rate at the aggregate level, the security it offers on the individual level is negligible (cf. chap. 9). In populations of European origin, the simplest methods (withdrawal, condom, diaphragm) are practiced with an average effectiveness of 95%. Their effectiveness can even reach 98% or 99% after the birth of the last child wanted (contraception for stopping births), as the study cited above showed; thus they nearly match the more "modern" methods such as the IUD or contraceptive pill, whose effectiveness is about 99% to 99.5%.

Finally, table 8.3 also includes some "continuation rates" for the modern methods (knowledge of these rates for the others are much poorer). As mentioned above, these rates must also be taken into account in judging the effectiveness of a method. What they show, in effect, is the degree of physical or psychological acceptability; for modern methods, with very high theoretical effectiveness, the estimate of the continuation rate is more important than counting the very few failures "of the method." Note that continuation rates recorded for mass family planning are usually lower than for single clinics. We may think that the other methods do not have higher continuation rates, but the cases where use is ended by an unwanted pregnancy are probably taken into account, at least partially, in the calculation of clinical failure rates.

Induced Abortion

With or without a contraceptive method, an undesired pregnancy may occur, and in this situation the woman may consider the possibility of abortion. The case of abortion is radically different from that of contraception, since it *increases*, rather than reduces, the degree of exposure to the risk of conception. That is, a woman carrying a pregnancy to term spends, on the average, 11 months in a nonsusceptible period of amenorrhea when there is breast-feeding; the amount of time is even longer if she breast-feeds her child. If she interrupts her pregnancy, the idle period is reduced to 4 or 5 months, and she is thus exposed sooner to the risk of a new conception.

Potter (1971, ref. 442) estimates that the number of induced abortions necessary to avert one live birth, in the absence of accompanying contraception, is 2.5 when the total period of amenorrhea associated with a live birth is about 20 months (long breast-feeding); with no breast-feeding, the number of abortions necessary would be just under 2. The more efficient the accompanying contraception, the nearer an abortion comes to averting one live birth (see Williams and Pullum 1975, ref. 403b).

In the models, induced abortion can be assimilated with spontaneous abortion for analyzing the length of the associated period of amenorrhea and the general functioning of the process. But instead of having the risk of abortion increase with age, or distributing it unequally among women, the assumption made is that after a certain number of live births some women will turn systematically to induced abortion in cases of unwanted pregnancies. That is, turning to abortion is considered here to be closer to the behavior of contraception for stopping births than to that of contraception for spacing.

Induced abortion may also be treated as an additional pregnancy outcome competing with the other outcomes, especially with spontaneous abortion (Potter et al. 1975, ref. 402b).

Sterilization

The distinction is even clearer in the case of sterilization, which is most often irreversible; from the individual's point of view, at least, reversibility is never certain. It is thus a question of ending reproduction, a decision that also depends heavily on the number of children already born.

In developed countries, where fertility is already low, sterilizations may also be performed for medical reasons (in a broad sense). For example, in the United States menopause was artificially induced in a large number of women even before the multiplication of sterilizations aimed specifically at limiting births. But since 1965 the total number of sterilizations has increased rapidly: at the end of 1973, 23% of American couples in which the woman was 15 to 44 years of age had undergone a surgical operation making them sterile; in 71% of these cases the operation was done for the purpose of contraception (W. Pratt [National Center for Health Statistics], "The practice of Sterilization in the United States: Preliminary Findings from the 1973 National Survey of Family Growth." Annual meeting of the P.A.A., Seattle, April 1975).

Sterilizations are infrequent, however, at early ages. This is why, in many high-fertility countries, sterilizations have little effect on total fertility: very often only couples aged 35 years and more, who already have 4 or 5 children, agree to be sterilized. In such cases the potential for averted births would be lower than expected.

The Demographic Effectiveness of Birth Control

The effect of birth control on natality or fertility may be defined in a simple way from a theoretical or modeling point of view: it is the number of births averted owing to use of a family planning method. In practice—in a real population—the concept is not so simple, since one is never sure what the behavior of users would have been if the method had not been available to them. There are many reasons for this uncertainty, the most important being that the population of family planning "acceptors" is never completely similar to that of "nonacceptors".

Let us consider the case of a family planning program and quickly examine some methods of evaluating its demographic impact. A distinction must be made between direct methods and indirect methods.

Direct methods are based solely on observed data.
   (*a*) Comparison between fertility before and after the program's inception
      M1. in the entire population (changes in reproduction rates, or age-specific fertility rates)
      M2. among acceptors (whose fertility both before and after the program must then be known)
   (*b*) Comparison between fertility of acceptors and of other groups
      M3. comparison with the entire population
      M4. comparison with another sample of the population
      M5. comparison with a sample having the same initial characteristics (age, parity, social category, etc.)
      M6. method of correlations (multivariate analysis): starting from a sample of acceptors and a sample of nonacceptors, with information about their sociodemographic characteristics, one investigates whether being an acceptor or not is correlated with the level of fertility, when other variables are "controlled."
Indirect methods require supplementary hypotheses on what fertility would have been in the absence of the program.
   (*c*) Methods of "demographic projections": one calculates the number of births that would occur in coming years if fertility were to remain at the same level, then compares this figure with the actual number of births
      M7. comparison for the entire population
      M8. comparison for the group of acceptors
   (*d*) Method of the calculation of "births averted"
      M9. One calculates first the "number of years of protection" acquired by the woman who starts using a certain method, then estimates the number of potential births she thus averts (e.g., an IUD insertion = 2.5 years of protection = 0.7 averted births).

Despite their "rational" character and their relative simplicity, these methods are far from providing indisputable answers to the question raised. Some examples of the problems involved are as follows.

Methods M1 and M2 (comparison over time): the idea that nothing in the population under study has changed *except* for the appearance of a family planning program is too naive. Fertility can be affected, independently of the program, if age at marriage or the behavior of couples changes, even among "nonacceptors." It is thus difficult to evaluate the specific role of the program.

Method M2 (fertility of acceptors): *previous* fertility of acceptors is often quite high (this is why they are acceptors); but, since they had enough motivation to become acceptors, would they not have reduced their fertility in any case (for example, by resorting to abortion)? Moreover, there are many "postpartum" programs. In these cases, when computing the fertility of the women during the 5 years preceding acceptance, one obtains a particularly high value because this period necessarily includes at least one pregnancy. The five following years, on the other hand, begin with a period of postpartum sterility.

Methods M3 and M4 (comparison with other samples): the characteristics of acceptors are often very different from those of the rest of the population— the former may be older and more fertile, but also more motivated. Thus care must be taken in comparisons.

Methods M5 and M6 are therefore preferable, since the comparison takes different sociodemographic variables into account.

Methods M7 and M8 (projections) are subject to the same criticisms as M1 and M2.

Method M9 (births averted) often leads to an over-optimistic estimate, since one does not know whether the methods prescribed are effectively and correctly used.

The use of models can be particularly useful for estimation by indirect methods. Several examples are given in the next chapter, and fuller treatments can be found by referring to section 2.32 of the Bibliography.

9

Models for the Study of Fertility

At the same time that the concepts discussed in the first six chapters were emerging and being refined, the idea of aggregating them to reconstitute the standard variables of demographic analysis (age-specific fertility rates, mean number of children, etc.) took shape. The first efforts attempted to completely formalize the process—that is, to express the desired indexes mathematically (and to establish general properties) from the distributions of the basic components. It soon became evident that this could not be fully carried out: in the most general case, when the parameters vary with age, with the number of births, and from one woman to another, when contraception is taken into account, the process becomes too complex to be fully expressed mathematically. Hence, various methods of simulation, either at a "macro" or a "micro" level, have been called into play.

Mathematical Models

As early as 1953, Henry worked on the problem of the algebraic formalization of the family-building process (ref. 285), which he was to develop more completely in three articles appearing in 1957 and 1961 (refs. 282, 283, 284). Leaving aside permanent sterility—assumed to occur at the same age in all couples—Henry defined three fundamental functions:

$p(x)$ = fecundability at age x;
$v(x)$ = probability that a conception (occurring at age x) will end in a live birth (or, "proportion of v-conceptions");
$K(x, g)$ = probability that a woman having conceived at age x will still be in the nonsusceptible state at age $x + g$ ($K = 0$ for $g > G$).

All three functions express a "risk" whose intensity is a function of the woman's age—not of the duration of marriage. This choice was dictated by the observations available from noncontracepting populations, where fertility was mostly a function of age. Thus the model was not applicable to contracepting populations.

These risks are assumed to be identical for all women, given equal age.

If there were no "nonsusceptible period," the number of conceptions (in a cohort with a size equal to one) would be at each moment equal to $p(x)$. Because of the existence of the nonsusceptible periods, the number of women who cannot be fertilized at a given moment must be removed from the number "at risk"; hence follows the fundamental equation:

$$C(x) = p(x)\left[1 - \int_0^G C(x - g) K(x - g, g)dg\right]. \tag{1}$$

This is an integral equation that cannot be explicitly solved. Nevertheless, it is possible to study the general form of its solutions, as Henry did in his 1957 article. The K function was actually split into two parts: K_A for the distribution of durations of the nonsusceptible period after a spontaneous abortion; and K_V for the distribution of durations of the nonsusceptible period after a live birth.

Proceeding with his theoretical study, Henry then calculated the cumulative number of conceptions from age at marriage (x_0) to some age x, the family size (number of live-born children) at that age, and the age-specific fertility rates; by doing the same calculations for the births of each order, he could make a detailed study of the successive intervals between births, in relation to the fertility rates. Some results Henry obtained using this method will be given later in this chapter.

For numerical applications, the formulas were of course converted to discrete notation, as I have done in Appendix A.

In a later article (1964, ref. 098), Henry took into account a double heterogeneity for fecundability and intrauterine mortality (by assuming the two distributions to be independent, which is—as we have seen—probably not a realistic hypothesis). But this model is not comparable to the preceding ones, since it is limited to the study of the interval between marriage and first birth.

Independently of Henry, but at the same time, Dandekar (1955, ref. 279a) used the theory of combinatorial analysis: instead of establishing recurrent formulas, he split a given period of time into possible combinations of nonsusceptible periods and delays to conception in order to derive a probability distribution of numbers of births for that period. In this case the formulation is necessarily discrete, and the time scale adopted is the month, since fecundability is defined as a monthly probability. In this very simplified model, intrauterine mortality was not taken into account, the nonsusceptible period was of fixed duration, and fecundability was constant and homogenous.

This model has been developed by numerous authors (Basu, Brass, Potter, Singh, Dharmadhikari, etc.), and it opened the way to the use of the theory of "renewal processes," especially Markov chains and semi-Markovian processes. In this theory, one defines a set of possible states and probabilities of transition from one state to another: counting the number of events is done by counting the number of transitions between states.

In the first model of this type, Perrin and Sheps (1964, ref. 303) postulated five states:

S_0: fertilization possible,
S_1: pregnancy,
S_2: postpartum sterility associated with a miscarriage,
S_3: postpartum sterility associated with a stillbirth,
S_4: postpartum sterility associated with a live birth.

Each woman enters the process via state S_0, moves after some months into state S_1, and from there into one of the other three states; after this, she returns to S_0. In the general theory of Markovian renewal processes, homogenous for external time, the time spent in each state is a random variable, whose distribution function can depend on both the current state and the following one: for example, the duration of pregnancy (S_1) is a function of the outcome of the pregnancy—that is, the nature of the following state (S_2, S_3, or S_4). But the distributions do not depend on total time elapsed: they can thus depend neither on age nor on the duration of marriage. This is the first limitation of the method.

Sheps and Menken (1973, ref. 313), however, have tried to remove this restriction, at least partially, notably by studying the effect of a discontinuity in one of the parameters. In this same work, they also take into account variable durations of postpartum sterility (from one woman, or one birth, to the next) and heterogenous fecundability.

The second limitation results from the fact that most of the formulas are established for the stationary case—that is, supposing an infinite time frame. In practice, convergence toward the stationary state is rapid enough for the model to give satisfactory results for that part of the reproductive period when the functions vary little, that is, between 20 and 35 years of age. However, it is impossible to describe periods when fecundity increases or decreases.

One of the great advantages of this method is that it lets one calculate not only the expected values of the various events studied, but also the *moments* of various orders—which were not examined at all by Henry. Let me also mention that certain extensions of the method are possible: modification of the distribution function at each return to a given state (essentially S_0) or modification of the probabilities of transition with time spent in a state ("internal time"). An overview of the results already obtained and the possible extensions may be found in an article by Sheps, Menken, and Radick (1969, ref. 314).

New developments have also appeared more recently. For example, Das Gupta (1973, ref. 279*b*) has extended the Perrin-Sheps model by taking into account three states of nursing (regular, irregular, absent), and infant mortality.

Simulation Models

The first group of simulation methods is close to the techniques described above. One begins with the mathematical formulation, but instead of solving it completely proceeds "step by step," deriving month by month the desired distributions from the ones obtained the month before. These are called macrosimulations.

The structure of the Fermod model, developed by Potter and Sakoda (1966, ref. 306; 1967, ref. 307), is as follows. A cohort of women is distributed, month by month, into various classes according to parity attained and status (susceptible to being fertilized, pregnant, or in postpartum period). In this way, "waiting lines" are established and managed so that women exit after a certain number of months. An example of the results obtained will be given later. This model is close to Henry's models in their discontinuous version.

But all reference to age is omitted; instead, fecundability (alone) becomes a function of birth order and can also undergo discontinuous modifications for certain marriage durations. The goal in this case is to elaborate a model applicable to the study of family-building in a contracepting population, which assumes that contraceptive effectiveness can be modified over time as the family "plan" unfolds.

Recently Bongaarts has proposed the application of the "system analysis" technique to the reproduction process (1975, ref. 275). As in the Markovian approach, one defines possible states and calculates the number of transitions from one state to another during each unit of time. But this number is calculated step by step, from the a priori distributions of times spent in the various states (time to conception, duration of nonsusceptible periods). These distributions are defined algebraically rather than numerically, so they can be made dependent on age or other parameters that vary during the process. The method is thus very flexible, except for taking heterogeneity into account.

Tietze and Bongaarts have given a good example of the use of this method for comparing contraception and induced abortion (1975, ref. 448).

Beginning in 1964, the diffusion of the "Monte Carlo method" gave rise to a series of models using the principle of *microsimulation*: for example, Hyrenius (1964), Ridley and Sheps (1966), Jacquard (1967), Lombardo (1968), Barrett (1969), Venkatacharya (1969), Horvitz et al. (1969), and Holmberg

(1970) (see references in section 1.4 of the bibliography). In this method each individual's history is simulated experimentally through random drawings repeated at each stage and for each possible event. Thus it is necessary neither to formulate explicitly the several conditional distributions nor to make an exhaustive list beforehand of all possible states. The model can therefore be richer; however, it introduces a "random error" that can be reduced only through the use of large "samples," a fact which leads to a substantial increase in computer time.

The extraordinary versatility of microsimulation permits it to approximate reality better than other methods. The list of possible events may be: marriage, widowhood, divorce, remarriage; death; permanent sterility; conception, under various hypotheses of contraceptive effectiveness according to the desired size and spacing for the family; intrauterine mortality. The various probabilities may be functions of age, duration of marriage, or birth order.

The possible applications are limitless. However, it is not necessary to start off by building a complex, intricate model; rather, it is better to keep the model's complexity within the limits required for each type of application. Furthermore, because of *data lacks*, the promise of microsimulation has been only partially realized.

After this theoretical presentation of the various models, for which a more complete list of references will be found in section 1.4 of the Bibliography, we move to a summary of some of the results that have been already obtained.

Some Theoretical Results Obtained by Henry

Although it would be impossible to summarize three very comprehensive articles in a few lines, it is still useful to mention here some of Henry's results that occasionally seem to have been forgotten.

Let us first consider the situation at the beginning of marriage. If $C(x)$ is the number of conceptions during month x (its formula having been given above), then the cumulated number of conceptions from marriage (at age x_0) to age x would be

$$Q(x) = \int_{x_0}^{x} C(\xi)d\xi$$

and the cumulative number of live births at the same age x

$$E(x) = \int_{x_0}^{x-g_0} v(\xi)C(\xi)d\xi,$$

where $v(\xi)$ is the proportion of V-conceptions at age ξ_1 and g_0 the duration of pregnancy for a live birth.

During the first years of marriage, the fertility rate,

$$\frac{Q(x)}{x - x_0}$$

may be subject to errors of interpretation. If we assume $p(x)$ and $K(x, g)$ to be *independent of age* x, which is justified, for example, over the interval of ages 20 to 30 years, and in the absence of premarital conceptions, the above fertility rate may be expressed as follows:

$$\frac{Q(x)}{x - x_0} = \frac{a}{x - x_0} + b + \frac{D(x - x_0)}{x - x_0}$$

with

$$a = b^2 \frac{\bar{g}^2 + \sigma_g^2}{2}$$

and

$$b = \frac{p}{1 + \bar{g}p}$$

It thus appears as the sum of a constant term, a hyperbolic term, and a damped oscillatory function.

The hyperbolic term is present because at the beginning of marriage the "mean rate of conception" always decreases, at first quite rapidly, since entry into observation (i.e., at marriage) corresponds to a unique situation: no woman is in a nonsusceptible period (we have excluded by hypothesis the existence of premarital conceptions).

Another consequence is to accentuate apparent fertility, at ages where marriages are the most frequent, when one calculates a rate of conception in a cohort of newly married women without regard for age at marriage. (These two effects should not be confused with the selection effect appearing in a cohort that is heterogeneous with respect to fecundability, and has been described in chap. 3.)

For live births (or v-conceptions), the decrease does not exist: the mean rate rises rapidly from zero to a maximum, somewhat higher than its asymptotic value. The index is thus more reliable for measuring fertility at the beginning of marriage.

In the two 1961 articles, Henry devoted an important place to the study of intervals between births and to relations between them and the basic functions, or fertility rates.

Let us consider a cohort of women (of size 1) who have conceived at an age x_0 and are terminating their nonsusceptible period at age $x_0 + g$.

Let $R(x)$ be the number who have not yet conceived at age x. $R(x)$ is simply an exponential such that

$$dR(x) = - p(x)R(x)dx,$$

from which, setting,

$$P(x) = \int_0^x p(t)dt,$$

we obtain

$$R(x) = \exp\left[-P(x) + P(x_0 + g)\right].$$

For these women, the mean duration of exposure to risk, u_g (or "mean time to conception"), is equal to

$$u_g = \frac{-\int_{x_0+g}^{\omega} (x - x_0 - g)dR(x)}{1 - R(\omega)},$$

ω standing for the upper age limit of fecundity.

As for mean interval between two conceptions, it equals the sum $g + u_g$. Let $h(g)$ be the probability density of g; the mean interval is

$$\bar{i}_c = \frac{\int_0^{\omega - x_0} (g + u_g) h(g)dg}{\int_0^{\omega - x_0} h(g)dg}.$$

In the case where p, v, and K are independent of age, and for ages sufficiently far away from the end of fecund life, ω, we find the simple expression

$$\bar{i}_c = \bar{g} + \frac{1}{p},$$

$\bar{g}$ signifying the mean of the distribution of nonsusceptible periods. In this case, it is also possible to calculate the mean interval between two v-conceptions, and thus between two live births:

$$\bar{i}_v = \frac{1}{v}\left(\bar{g} + \frac{1}{p}\right).$$

In order to calculate age-specific fertility rates, it is necessary to fix the intervals' position with respect to some age group. Let δ be the age interval considered (e.g., 20 to 25 years, or 20 to 30 years).

An interval between two births may fall completely within δ, and would then be called an "interior interval"; it may also cross one of the two bounds of δ, and in this case it is called "straddling." The basic functions are assumed to be independent of age, for a period somewhat wider than δ on both sides. Let $\bar{i}$ be the mean interval between live births (in the period considered),

$\bar{y}$ the mean length of a straddling interval,

$\bar{j}$ the mean of an interior interval,

k the number of women involved, and

n_i the number of children borne by a woman i during the interval δ.

Henry shows first of all that the fertility rate *for later fertile women* is equal to

$$
f = \frac{\sum_1^k n_i}{k\delta} = \frac{\sum_i^k n_i}{\bar{y}\frac{k}{2} + j\sum(n_i - 1) + \bar{y}\frac{k}{2}}.
$$

In other words, $1/f$ is a weighted mean of intervals that have their beginning or end in the period δ, with interior intervals counted twice.

If γ stands for the coefficient of variation (standard deviation over the mean) of the distribution of intervals after a conception, $\bar{y}$ and j are shown as

$$
j = \bar{i}\left(1 - \frac{\bar{i}\gamma^2}{\delta - \bar{i}}\right)
$$

and

$$
\bar{y} \simeq \bar{i}(1 + \gamma^2).
$$

One must note that $j < \bar{i}$, and $\bar{y} > \bar{i}$; in other words, neither the mean of the straddling intervals nor that of the closed intervals equals the overall mean of the intervals.

Some Theoretical Results Obtained by Sheps and Menken

Since the series of articles by Henry, the most noteworthy effort at synthesis is that of Sheps and Menken (1973, ref. 313); several of their results have already been mentioned, especially in chapter 3. Some others of general interest will be given here.

As Henry did, Sheps and Menken have thoroughly analyzed distributions of various intervals between events (for example, between two successive births). Let μ be the mean, σ^2 the variance, and $\mu^{(n)}$ the nth-order moment of an interval. Usually these intervals are called "closed" to distinguish them from other types of intervals, such as an "open" interval, a period between the last event preceding a survey and the date of the survey; and a "straddling" interval, which is a closed interval spanning the date of the survey (or any other fixed point independent of the event being studied).

For the first (open), the mean and variance have the well-known forms

$$
EY_0 = \frac{\mu^{(2)}}{2\mu} = \tfrac{1}{2}\left(\mu + \frac{\sigma^2}{\mu}\right)
$$

$$
\text{Var } Y_0 = \frac{\mu^{(3)}}{3\mu} - \frac{[\mu^{(2)}]^2}{4\mu^2}.
$$

For the second (straddling), the formulas are

$$EY_S = \mu + \frac{\sigma^2}{\mu} = 2EY_0$$

$$\text{Var } Y_S = \frac{\mu^{(3)}}{\mu} - \frac{[\mu^{(2)}]^2}{\mu^2}.$$

As for the actual interval between births, Sheps and Menken calculate it as a function of its components, especially in the case where these components are homogenous and constant: fecundability equal to p; rate of intrauterine mortality equal to α; total duration of the nonsusceptible period equal to $(m - 1)$ for a live birth and $(w - 1)$ for a spontaneous abortion, in the discrete case; and no sterility.

The mean interval between births is expressed as follows:

$$\mu = \frac{1}{(1 - \alpha)p} + m + \frac{w\alpha - 1}{1 - \alpha}$$

or

$$\mu = \frac{Gp + (1 - p)}{(1 - \alpha)p}$$

with $G = m(1 - \alpha) + w\alpha$ (mean nonsusceptible period).

The limit value of the fertility rate is, under these hypotheses, equal to the inverse of the interval between births.

An Example of "Macrosimulation": FERMOD (by Potter and Sakoda)

We have already reviewed some *theoretical* results obtained by Henry. His study was completed by numerical applications, which allowed him to study the variation of fecundability with age.

This aspect of the question disappears in the models which aim at studying the effects of contraception. Fertility, in this case, is no longer a function of age but of the duration of marriage or, rather, of the number of children already born, through family planning and contraceptive effectiveness. This is the case in the FERMOD model of Potter and Sakoda (1966, ref. 306; 1967, ref. 307) which has been mentioned above. The authors distinguish three possible outcomes for a pregnancy: (1) spontaneous abortion (18% of the cases): associated nonsusceptible period $3 + 1$ months; (2) stillbirth (2% of the cases): associated nonsusceptible period $9 + 3$ months; and (3) live birth (80% of the cases): associated nonsusceptible period $9 + g$ months, g having a fixed distribution and a mean of 3.5 months.

With respect to fecundability, the "natural" value is assumed to be constant (for example, 0.28), but its "residual" value depends on birth order, as a function of the parents' "family plan." This plan is defined by: a final goal in terms of live births (three); desired intervals between births (one, two, or three years); and the effectiveness of the contraceptive method, either for spacing births (0.90) or after the goal has been reached (0.95 or 0.99). The output variables are the following: distribution of families by final size; mean, standard deviation, and skewness of this distribution; mean and standard deviation of the intervals between marriage and birth of order n.

Table 9.1 gives a sample of the results obtained.

Table 9.1. Proportion of Couples Having More Children Than Expected

| Natural Fecundability | Contraceptive Effectiveness when Limiting | | | |
| | 0.95 | | 0.99 | |
	Close Spacing (1)	Wide Spacing (2)	Close Spacing (1)	Wide Spacing (2)
0.50	0.975	0.958	0.527	0.479
0.28	0.869	0.815	0.336	0.289
0.14	0.620	0.546	0.177	0.147
0.07	0.343	0.292	0.081	0.067

SOURCE: Potter and Sakoda 1967 (ref. 307; p. 323).
NOTE: Desired family size = 3 children.
(1) One year from marriage to first birth, two years between successive births. Contraceptive effectiveness for spacing: 90%.
(2) Two years from marriage to first birth, three years between successive births. Contraceptive effectiveness for spacing: 90%.

The strength of these models, then, is their ability to treat cohorts and thus to calculate types of indexes (here, the proportions who exceed their goal, according to various "individual" criteria), which in overall analysis is not possible. Moreover, these results can be linked with results valid at the overall level, as the next example will show.

An Example of Microsimulation (Jacquard and Bodmer)

Microsimulation models permit another step in the increasing complexity of the process; this may be done in two directions: either by elaboration of the physiological hypotheses (for example, by reinserting some variation of natural fecundability with age), or by being closer to realistic demographic conditions, by taking into account deaths and entries into, and dissolution of, unions; the model could even be integrated into a more general model of population change. Moreover, the method allows the analysis of variance.

The parameters of the Jacquard and Bodmer model (1967, ref. 295; 1968 ref. 274) are the following: (1) monthly probabilities of marriage, widowhood, death, and divorce (the last three by duration of marriage), from 15 to 45 years; (2) natural fecundability as a function of age (increasing from 15 to 20 years, constant from 20 to 30 years at the 0.25 level, and decreasing from

30 to 45 years); (3) a constant rate of intrauterine mortality (25%); (4) distributions of the nonsusceptible period according to pregnancy outcome; and (5) for contraception, the number of children desired, preferred intervals between births, and levels of contraceptive effectiveness for spacing or limiting births.

The output variables are: (1) mean ages of women at the time of conceptions of various orders; (2) mean intervals between successive conceptions; (3) variance of these intervals; (4) number of conceptions of various orders by year of age.

As in the preceding model, it is thus possible to obtain individual rates of success or failure. For example, when three is the desired number of children, the authors obtained the following proportions of those exceeding this number: 49% with contraception for limiting births 95% effective (with spacing contraception, 90% and desired interval of 3 years); and 18% with contraception for limiting births 99% effective (same hypotheses as above for spacing).

The second proportion is close to the result obtained by Potter and Sakoda for a fecundability of between 0.14 and 0.28 (with 15% and 29%, respectively, exceeding their desired family size), but the first proportion is lower (55% and 81% exceeding for the same fecundabilities); the discrepancy probably results from the inclusion of dissolutions of unions.

In the aggregate, the results may be translated into reproduction rates: one can thus see overall effectiveness of contraception. The hypotheses on natural fertility retained by the authors lead to a net reproduction rate greater than 4. This value is probably too high; one possible explanation might be that the progressive decrease in fecundability with age is not rapid enough to compensate for the absence of sterility before 45 years of age: at 35 years of age, as we have seen, about 16% of all women are already permanently sterile.

If all couples wanted three children and practiced contraception with moderate effectiveness (70% for spacing and 90% for limiting), the net reproduction rate would be about 2; with a high effectiveness (90% for spacing and 99% for limiting), the rate would fall to 1.3.

Thus, in the aggregate, contraception plays an important role in two ways: when average contraceptive effectiveness is low, failures keep total fertility at a level higher than that desired by individuals; but when effectiveness is very high, contraception can keep people from reaching their goal by delaying a conception until a time when it is no longer possible (due to separation, sterility, low fecundability).

Remaining Problems

All the models result in some dispersion of final family size. This dispersion is the consequence of the various probabilities used—for fecundability, duration of the nonsusceptible period, age at marriage, or contraceptive effectiveness. An essential factor of dispersion remains to be considered: the heterogeneity of real cohorts with respect to the various risks mentioned.

It is entirely possible to manipulate heterogeneous cohorts in a micro-simulation process, since the final result is obtained by addition of individual histories, treated one by one. In the other types of models, one could, if necessary, incorporate the dispersion of one parameter by mixing several homogeneous cohorts, but taking account of more than one source of dispersion would once again pose the problem of *conditional* distributions.

Bodmer and Jacquard had the idea of comparing the variance of final family size yielded by their model (under the hypotheses of natural fertility) with the *real* variance observed among (strictly noncontracepting) Hutterite women. The latter is *two and a half times higher* than the former, which shows that homogeneous models are far from reflecting the heterogeneity of real cohorts.

In another discussion of this point (Jacquard and Leridon 1974, ref. 296), I have shown that taking a distribution of fecundability among women into account is enough to obtain a variance of intervals between births, or of the distribution of the final number of children, compatible with observations of natural fertility. This result may seem paradoxical, since I have also mentioned the existence of dispersion in the risk of intrauterine mortality and the duration of the nonsusceptible period. For the former, postulating independent distributions of fecundability and intrauterine mortality would certainly be redundant: the two concepts are so closely linked that a woman with a high risk of spontaneous abortion is also likely to have low fecundability. As for the nonsusceptible period, the practice is to use an identical distribution for all women, at least those of the same age, and to have an independent probability drawing at each live birth. The empirical distribution used thus includes both the *internal* variance (for the successive births of one woman) and the variance *among* women. This solution is forced upon us, since we do not know the respective contributions of these two variances and we have no grounds for combining independent distributions.

All this raises the problem of evaluating a model's adequacy. What seems necessary in this respect is an analysis of variance (on intervals, or the distribution of the number of children), since it is easy to build a model yielding simply suitable *means*. The analysis of intervals between births grouped both by birth order and by final family size also furnishes, as we have seen, an indicator that is especially sensitive to changes in the parameters with woman's age.

The SIMULA Model

In chapter 7, a microsimulation model (SIMNAT) was used to study the possible range of levels of natural fertility and to evaluate the role of each parameter in this distribution. This was a version, without birth control, of a more general program, which I derived from the Jacquard and Bodmer model in an attempt to define the "optimum structure "of such a model. Considering what I have presented up to this point, it seems that the model should have the following structure.

Let us first deal with the physiological variables. Puberty is assumed to be acquired before marriage but, from 15 to 20 years of age, fecundability rises from some initial (greater than zero) value to its maximum level. This maximum level varies from one woman to another and is defined at the time of the woman's marriage (by drawing from an approximately normal, or from a beta, distribution). The decline of fecundability at the end of the reproductive period is related to the age of onset of sterility. Let S_x be this age; fecundability drops from its maximum level to zero over an interval $(S_x - D)$ to S_x. In accordance with the results shown in Appendix A, D has been set equal to 12.5 years.

Intrauterine mortality is the same for all women, but it varies with age. The distribution of the nonsusceptible period associated with a pregnancy is, of course, a function of the outcome of the pregnancy. In the case of a live birth, the numerical values chosen can represent the effect both of the duration (or frequency) of breast-feeding and of infant mortality. In the present version, the duration of the nonsusceptible period is a function neither of mother's age nor of pregnancy rank, but it would be easy to introduce a multiplier to take these into account. Finally, the age of onset of permanent sterility is defined at the beginning of each individual simulation. It would be both possible and desirable to add a risk to each pregnancy to the risk caused by aging: this could be accomplished by including an additional drawing at the end of each pregnancy.

Let us move now to behavioral variables. The first, already taken into account in the SIMNAT version, is of course age at marriage, defined at the beginning of each simulation. The SIMULA version includes risks of widowhood, divorce, and remarriage as well as the risk of the woman's death. These are monthly probabilities, very costly in computer time, which will be replaced by drawings at the beginning of each "segment" of marital life.

Family planning is the result of the choice of the number of children desired, the effectiveness of contraception for limiting births (once the desired number is attained), the desired spacing between births, and the effectiveness of contraception for spacing.

As an example, here is a case similar to those analyzed by Jacquard, which attempts to measure the effect of contraception in a modern, Western type of population, characterized by low permanent celibacy (6%), mean age at marriage (for women) of between 21 and 22 years, risk of divorce of about 12%, and low mortality. As for physiological variables, fecundability is 0.25, risk of spontaneous abortion 25%, and the postpartum nonsusceptible period equal to 10 months on the average (thus corresponding to a period of breast-feeding lasting 1 to 1.5 years). In this example sterility is not taken into account before the age of 45 years.

The consequence of the hypothesis of long breast-feeding is that fertility does not reach a very high level, even in the absence of contraception; according to table 7.3, fertility would be about one-third higher with no breast-feeding. But this seemed to be a more realistic point of comparison than a situation in which fertility would attain a level never observed in any population.

Some results of the simulation are given in the last column of table 9.2. I propose comparison with a situation where all couples desire three children, and to obtain this objective practice contraception with a relatively low effectiveness: 70% for spacing births (desired interval 3 years), 90% after the birth of the third child.

Table 9.2.   Comparison between Fertility Levels in a Noncontracepting Population (European Type, Low Mortality, Widespread Breast-feeding) and Fertility Levels in the Same Population When Practicing Contraception with a Low Effectiveness

	With Contraception (1)	No Contraception
Distribution of 100 Married Women by Final Number of Children		
Number fewer than desired (0,1,2)	5	3
Number equal to desired (3)	28	5
Number greater than desired (4 and more)	67	92
Mean Number of Children		
Per married woman	4.04	8.37
Per woman	3.84	7.86
Net reproduction rate	1.8	3.7
Mean age of childbearing (years)	29.5	31.6
Mean intervals (months)		
Marriage to 1st birth	25.4	14.7
1st to 2d birth	32.6	27.0
2d to 3d birth	32.2	25.3

NOTE: Desired family size = 3 children.
(1) Effectiveness of contraception: spacing = 70%; limiting = 90%.

It appears that in these two cases a wide majority of women have more children than they desire: 92% in the absence of contraception, and 67% even when some method is used. In terms of the mean number of children the gap is more significant, since it drops from 8.4 (per married woman) to 4.0. The result is a decrease in the net reproduction rate, from 3.7 to 1.8, which shows once again that contraception practiced with a low effectiveness from the individual point of view can nonetheless have substantial demographic impact.

10

Overview

Having reached the end of this analysis, we can see that the two methods described—direct observation whenever possible, and study through models—have proved complementary. Some of the missing links in the chain of available observations can, in fact, often be supplied by the use of logical schemata. Let me now try to summarize the contents of the first six chapters.

I early emphasized the fact that fertilization is a process subject to many disorders; the failure rate is surely greater than 40% and may reach 65%.

The reproductive period, which "theoretically" has a mean length of 35 years (from puberty to menopause), actually is reduced to an average of 27–28 years.

Fertility is the result of the combination of several behavioral factors and physiological variables. I said that, under conditions of natural fertility, these behavioral factors are not modified by individual couples trying to regulate their fertility, but rather constitute the social norms to which couples conform (in a constant manner) all their lives. As to physiological factors, they work through the four fundamental components of natural fertility:

1. (Natural) *fecundability*, or monthly probability of conceiving for a susceptible woman, generally involves only recognizable pregnancies, that is, those that lead to a delay in menses noticed by the woman herself; it is about 30% at age 25. Including only conceptions which end in live births, we can determine effective fecundability to be about 20% to 25%. Fecundability differs from one woman to another, and its variance can be estimated approximately through the use of the distribution of "waiting time to conception," which increases with age between puberty and age 20 and probably diminishes beyond 30–35 years of age.

2. *Intrauterine mortality* is very high during the first 2 weeks of gestation (about 40%), but there it mingles with fecundability as defined above. After the first 2 weeks, 20% to 25% of the pregnancies still in progress are affected by intrauterine mortality. This estimate can be made only by the "life table"

method; it corresponds to a rate of about 10% to 15% from current (retrospective) observations.

Intrauterine mortality increases rapidly with age after age 30. This increase is found even for first-order conceptions; it may even be more rapid for these than for others. The distribution of risk among women can be estimated by analyzing the outcomes of successive pregnancies. This distribution can explain the very rapid increase in the risk of intrauterine death after each miscarriage (a doubling of the risk after the first miscarriage is often observed).

3. The *Postpartum nonsusceptible period* is equal, on the average, to the duration of postpartum amenorrhea, which depends directly on duration of lactation. An approximate relationship between the two periods is proposed in table 10.1.

Table 10.1.   Relation between the Duration of Lactation and the Nonsusceptible Period

Mean Duration of Lactation (Months)	Median Nonsusceptible Period (Months)
0	2
3	3
6	4 to 5
12	6 to 9
18	9 to 13
24	12 to 17

The effect of breast-feeding probably varies among populations, perhaps owing to differing sanitary conditions or nutrition; this is why *ranges* are given in table 10.1. The length of the nonsusceptible period also increases with the age of the woman. For example, then, in a population where breast-feeding is practiced for 12 to 18 months after childbirth, the mean interval between births is increased by 6 to 12 months.

4. *Permanent sterility* is acquired "spontaneously" (i.e., in a nonpathological manner) at ages varying among women. The distribution of the age of its onset is not well known. I have given only two estimates (both fairly old), by Vincent and by Henry. According to these authors, the proportion of women already sterile is about 3% at age 20, 6% at age 25, 10% at age 30, 16% at age 35, and 31% at age 40. It is possible, however, that higher proportions might be observed in populations with less favorable nutrition or sanitary conditions (indeed, some obvious examples of this are known). Under normal conditions, the risk of onset of permanent sterility seems to be independent of the number of children already born, although there is an additional risk associated with each confinement.

Combining all these variables leads to very different levels of fertility. The average final number of live births of a woman who marries at age 20, and remains in an unbroken union until age 45, can vary from 5 to 11. Marital fertility rates for ages 20 to 24, for example, vary from 280 to 550 births per 1,000 women per year.

Marriage conditions (age at marriage, frequency of divorce and of re-marriage after divorce or widowhood), combined with mortality conditions (frequency of widowhood), will also affect the final number of children. These two influences can be studied using models based on the four components. For example, I have proposed the following results:

1. The biological maximum for women remaining fecund and exposed to risk from their 15th to their 45th birthdays, and not breast-feeding their children, would be about 17 to 18 children.[1]

2. Taking into account a minimum level of sterility, and more realistic assumption on nuptiality (Asian or African type), the mean number would be around 13 children.[2]

3. In practice, since it is very rare for women in situations of natural fertility not to breast-feed their children at all, the observed average would not exceed 11 children.

4. At the opposite extreme, under conditions of early sterility, prolonged breast-feeding, and late marriage (i.e., around age 25), the average number might be around 4 children, even in a "natural fertility" situation.

We see, therefore, that fertility regulation can occur in various ways. This is why the intent of the last two chapters was to show the link that exists between situations of natural fertility and others: contraceptive practice, use of induced abortion, and voluntary sterilization. Including these variables in models thus brings them to their full effectiveness—and their full topicality.

1. An *average* result; some women would have up to 25 children, others "only" 10.
2. This would be approximately the case for a European or American woman who married at age 18 or 19.

Appendix A
Use of a
Model for
Studying
Birth Intervals
by Final
Family Size

I presented in chapter 7 two examples of networks of intervals between births grouped by birth order and final family size (figs. 7.2 and 7.3). These were for families practicing little or no birth control. A distinctive aspect of these networks is the large increase in the length of the last interval, for every final family size.

The occurrence of permanent sterility cannot be responsible for this increase, since by definition each woman is still fecund at the time of her last conception. The lengthening of the interval could result: from a rapid decrease in fecundability above a certain age; from a rapid increase in intrauterine mortality above a certain age; or from a lengthening of the postpartum nonsusceptible period.

We have seen from the detailed study of these factors that the three changes mentioned above are possible, and even probable. But these analyses were done without specifying final family size (most often on incomplete families), and thus they are not directly useful for our present discussion. Our task is to attempt to reconstruct, using specific hypotheses, a network similar to those of figures 7.2 and 7.3: some hypotheses will be accepted or rejected, according to the model's results. In consideration of the large number of parameters involved, it is not feasible to examine all the possibilities. The research will thus focus on the following question: *What pattern of fecundability with age, or of intrauterine mortality with age, leads to an increase in final intervals close to the one observed?*

Characteristic
Shape of a Network

Let me mention before proceeding further a simple method (from Henry) for getting an idea of the pattern of intervals, taking final family size into account, when the number of observations available does not allow us to construct the entire network. One must rearrange the data for *a group of* final sizes (for example, 8 children and over) and then calculate rank by rank the mean successive intervals, in two steps. (1) first the usual calculation of mean intervals between first and second births, between second and third births, and so on, up to the $(n - 4)^{th}$ or $(n - 3)^{rd}$ birth, n being the mean size of families in the group chosen (for example, 9); (2) then a *backward* calculation of mean intervals—between the last and next-to-last births, between next-to-last and second-to-last, and so on, until overlapping the previous series. If n (mean size) is not close to a whole number (for example, $n = 9.5$), intervals are placed on the graph as if the scale of birth orders were continuous.

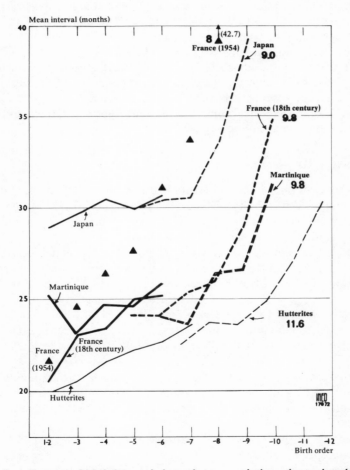

Fig. A.1.   Pattern of birth intervals in various populations (completed families of 8 or more children).

Since it seems that the last intervals corresponding to each final family size may be superimposed by simple translation (which my study will confirm), it is clear that the "mixture" of various family sizes carried out in this way retains the general form of each series. In the case where random fluctuations make the sketch of the complete network impossible, this is therefore a means of showing what I shall call the "characteristic shape" of the network.

Figure A.1 shows the characteristic shapes of networks mentioned in chapter 7, as well as the results of several other studies: a sample of women of Martinique, from the survey already cited (ref. 349); in this group, because of conditions specific to the Antilles, matrimonial status was not taken into account; the Hutterites (ref. 353), a sect living in the United States and refusing all contraception; French families, from a study connected with the 1954 census (unpublished data from INSEE). (The numerical data may be found in Appendix B, table B.3.)

Despite the considerable heterogeneity of these data, the curves still form regular tiers by final family size. Only the first half of the curve for modern French families is somewhat out of line, a consequence of the fact that, in these families the spacing of births—even in large families—is less the result of breast-feeding than of a minimum of contraception, the effectiveness of which may improve continuously with age.

Description of the Model Used

In his study of birth intervals, Henry had to limit himself to a single source of variability—fecundability—which was a function of age. Moreover, the nonsusceptible periods were always of the same duration (18 months), and intrauterine mortality was assumed to be zero.

The purposes here will be threefold: (1) to make the model more realistic by reintroducing intrauterine mortality and a distribution for the nonsusceptible period; (2) to compare the effects of a continuous increase in intrauterine mortality with age with those of a decrease in fecundability at the end of the reproductive period; (3) in order to make the general form of the network more explicit, to take into account a distribution of "entries into fertile life" (ages at marriage) and a distribution of "exits from fertile life" (ages at sterility).

The first two objectives will be reached by direct programming of the proper formulas, while the third will require the recombination of the results obtained for various ages at marriage and ages at the end of the reproductive period.

The notation is as follows. In general, a subscript i will refer to the *order* of the conception, and the subscripts j or k to a *time* elapsed or to an *age* (in quarters).

Let P_j be the fecundability during quarter j;

L_j the proportion of "V conceptions" (live births) among all conceptions of quarter j;

K_{j-k} the proportion of women who are still in a nonsusceptible status $(j - k)$ quarters after a conception;

S_{j-k} the proportion of women who are still in a nonsusceptible status $(j - k)$ quarters after a conception V;

T_{j-k} the proportion of women still in a nonsusceptible status $(j - k)$ quarters after a conception A.

The size of the cohort is set equal to 1. The subscript j (quarter) varies from O to F. The distribution S_{j-k} is limited to 10 quarters, and that of T_{j-k} to 1 quarter.

Let C_{ij} be the number of conceptions of order i during quarter j, and V_{ij} the number of V-conceptions of order i during quarter j.

C_{ij} and V_{ij} are calculated by means of doubly recurrent equations:

$$C_{ij} = P_j \left[\sum_{k=0}^{j-1} (C_{i-1,\,k} - C_{i,\,k}) - \sum_{k=j-10}^{j-1} C_{i-1,\,k} K_{j-k} \right]$$

for $i \geq 2$;

for $i = 1$, we use:

$$C_{1j} = P_j \left[1 - \sum_{k=0}^{j-1} C_{1k} \right]$$

And similarly,

$$V_{ij} = P_j L_j \left[\sum_{k=0}^{j-1} (V_{i-1,\,k} - V_{i,\,k}) - \sum_{k=j-10}^{j-1} V_{i-1,\,k} S_{j-k} - \frac{1 - L_{j-1}}{L_{j-1}} V_{i,\,j-1} T_1 \right]$$

with

$$V_{1j} = P_j L_j \left[1 - \sum_{k=0}^{j-1} V_{1,\,k} - \frac{1 - L_{j-1}}{L_{j-1}} V_{1,\,j-1} T_1 \right].$$

In this formula, the time-origin is the marriage (cohort of newly married women, size set equal to 1). For studying successive intervals, the time-distribution of conceptions following a conception occurring at a given age must be available. The probability that a conception, occurring during quarter t, will be followed by another during quarter j is

$$E_{t,j} = P_j L_j \left[1 - S_{j-t} - \sum_{k=t}^{j-1} E_{t,k} - \frac{1 - L_{j-1}}{L_{j-1}} T_1 E_{t,j-1} \right],$$

(setting $S_{j-t} = 0$ once $j - t > 10$).

We are now in a position to simultaneously take into account age at time of conception and rank of the conception. The final family size remains to be considered. For this, we must calculate the probability that a v-conception occurring during quarter t, will be followed by exactly m others during the woman's reproductive period. This probability is given again by a recurrent formula:

$$P_{m,t} = \sum_{j=t+1}^{F} E_{t,j} P_{m-1,j}.$$

The calculations of the V_{ij}'s, and then of the E_{tj}'s and P_{mt}'s, are done *independently*. Then the results obtained are combined to arrive at the desired intervals: the probability that there will be, during quarter j, a v-conception of order i and that this conception will be followed by exactly m others, is equal to

$$Z_j(i, m) = V_{ij} P_{mj}.$$

To obtain the distribution of v-conceptions, rank by rank, in families of final family size D, one need only apply the preceding formula to values of m such that: $m = D - i$.

The number of these families of final size D is equal to

$$N_D = \sum_{j=0}^{F} Z_j(i, D - i) = \sum_{j=0}^{F} V_{ij} P_{(D-i),j},$$

the result necessarily the same for each i.

The mean duration between marriage and the ith v-conception in families of final size D, is equal to

$$X_{(i, D)} = \frac{1}{N_D} \sum_{j=0}^{F} j Z_j(i, D - i).$$

The difference between the $X(i, D)$ for two successive orders i gives the desired intervals.

Numerical Values of Various Parameters

The analysis done by Henry showed that: (1) the mean values of fecundability or of the nonsusceptible period have little influence on the increase in the last interval; (2) this increase is proportional to the duration of the decrease in fecundability, which must be between 10 and 15 years; and (3) the distance between the various curves for various final family sizes depends on the degree of heterogeneity of the group with respect to fecundability and the nonsusceptible period.

As a result, the *homogeneity* assumed in the model does not affect the characteristic shape of the network but might vary the curves' spacing.

In my applications, I have taken point (2) above into account by assuming the decrease in fecundability to extend over 15 years (from 30 to 45 years of age).

I have adopted here the distributions of durations of the nonsusceptible period used by Henry in his other applications. Here are the values of the various parameters:

1. Proportion of women still not susceptible in quarter j among all women having had a V-conception in quarter k (S_{j-k}):

$j-k$:	0	1	2	3	4	5	6	7	8	9	10	$\geqslant 11$
S_{j-k}	1	1	1	1	0.856	0.822	0.789	0.722	0.500	0.211	0.044	0

2. Proportion of women still not susceptible in quarter j among all women having had an A conception in quarter k (T_{j-k}):

$j-k$:	0	1	$\geqslant 2$
T_{j-k}	1	0.90	0

3. Maximum final size of families for whom the succession of intervals is calculated (D_{max}): $D_{max} = 13$.

4. Length of the reproductive period (F) (from marriage to permanent sterility):

In quarters:	20	40	60	80	90
In years:	5	10	15	20	22.5

These values can be used to vary either age at marriage or age of sterility.

5. Fecundability—three hypotheses of variation with age: (*a*) constant (quarterly value = 0.50); (*b*) constant (0.578) until age 30, then decreasing linearly until age 45; (*c*) constant (0.833) until age 30, then decreasing linearly until age 45.

6. Intrauterine mortality—three hypotheses of variation with age: (*a*) constant (25%); (*b*) increasing, from 16% (at 22.5 years) to 50% (at 45 years); (*c*) increasing, from 16% (at 22.5 years) to 100% (at 45 years)

Table A.1 shows the five combinations of fecundability and intrauterine mortality chosen for study from among all possible combinations.

7. Permanent sterility; and

8. Age at marriage: The appropriate distributions will be given at the proper time.

Table A.1. Assumptions for Fecundability and Intrauterine Mortality

Code		\multicolumn{10}{c}{Age (in Years)}
		22.5	25	27.5	30	32.5	35	37.5	40	42.5	45
C_{15}	P_j	0.578	0.578	0.578	0.576	0.49	0.39	0.29	0.19	0.09	0.00
	L_j	0.75	0.75	0.75	0.75	0.75	0.75	0.75	0.75	0.75	0.75
C'	P_j	0.50	0.50	0.50	0.50	0.50	0.50	0.50	0.50	0.50	0.50
	L_j	0.840	0.826	0.806	0.777	0.740	0.690	0.616	0.460	0.230	0.00
C''	P_j	0.50	0.50	0.50	0.50	0.50	0.50	0.50	0.50	0.50	0.50
	L_j	0.840	0.826	0.806	0.777	0.740	0.686	0.619	0.561	0.520	0.50
C'_{15}	P_j	0.578	0.578	0.578	0.576	0.49	0.39	0.29	0.19	0.09	0.00
	L_j	0.840	0.826	0.806	0.777	0.740	0.690	0.616	0.460	0.230	0.00
P'_{15}	P_j	0.833	0.833	0.833	0.826	0.686	0.546	0.406	0.266	0.126	0.00
	L_j	0.840	0.826	0.806	0.777	0.740	0.690	0.616	0.460	0.230	0.00

NOTE: P_j = fecundability at age j; L_j = proportion of pregnancies (beginning at age j) ending in a live birth.

Effect of the Evolution of Fecundability and Intrauterine Mortality with Age

For the first applications of this model, I have taken the hypotheses adopted by Henry, that is: decreasing fecundability (from 0.50 to 0) in 10 years (model B_{10}) or in 15 years (model B_{15}); no intrauterine mortality; and nonsusceptible period constant and equal to 6 months. The results are shown

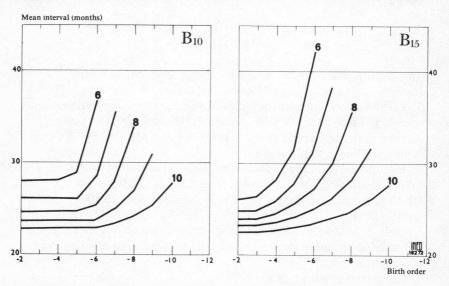

Fig. A.2. Birth intervals, by birth order and final size of family: Assumptions B_{10} and B_{15}.

in figure A.2. (The *numerical results* have not been reproduced here; they may be found in the French edition.)

The main difference between these and the real data (figs. 7.2 and 7.3) is the progressive enlargement of networks B_{10} and B_{15}: the increase of the last interval is inversely proportional to final family size in these cases.

Thus, in B_{15} the last interval is 10 months longer than the next to last in families of 6 children, and less than 2 months longer in families of 10 children.

To facilitate the comparisons, we will compute for each network (see table A.2): the increase (R_m) in the last interval in families with final size equal to the mean (m) of final sizes (with R_m determined by interpolation if m is not close to a whole number); the difference between the increase of the last interval in families of 6 children (R_6) and families of 10 children (R_{10}) as an index of the "widening of the fan"; and the difference between the interval from the first birth to the second birth in families of 6 children (I_6), and the same interval in families of 10 children as an index of the "spread" of the network.

In order to agree with the observed networks, R_m must be about 7 months and ($R_6 - R_{10}$) must be as small as possible (1–2 months); this is not the case for B_{10} or B_{15}.

Table A.2. Patterns of Birth Intervals (Model's Values and Actual Data)

Code	m	R_m	$R_6 - R_{10}$	D_m	I_m	$I_6 - I_{10}$
B_{10}	8.7	4.6	5.4	31.9	23.9	5.3
B_{15}	8.0	5.5	8.3	35.4	23.9	3.5
C_{15}	7.9	5.5	5.0	39.4	28.5	9.1
C'	8.2	4.7	1.9	36.7	28.6	9.5
C''	9.0	1.1	6.6	33.7	28.7	10.3
C'_{15}	7.4	6.7	3.5	39.6	27.6	8.2
P'_{15}	8.1	6.2	3.2	37.3	25.8	7.3
C^s_{15}	7.1	5.3	1.7	38.7	29.3	7.3
D^s_{15}	5.2	5.2	1.1	38.6	29.6	9.0
M^s_{15}	6.7	5.0	1.4	38.1	29.3	6.0
Actual data (Families of size 5 and more)						
Japan	7.2	7	2.0[b]	43	32	8.8
France (18th century)	8.1	7	1.6	38	25.5[a]	5.8[a]
Martinique	7.4	~8	—	~38	~28	—
Amish	8.0	~5	~9	~38	24[a]	6.8[a]

NOTE: m = mean of final family sizes; R_i = difference between last and next-to-last intervals in families of size i; D_i = length of last interval in families of size i; I_i = length of the interval between first and second births in families of size i.
[a] This value was computed for intervals between *second* and third births.
[b] $R_6 - R_{11}$.

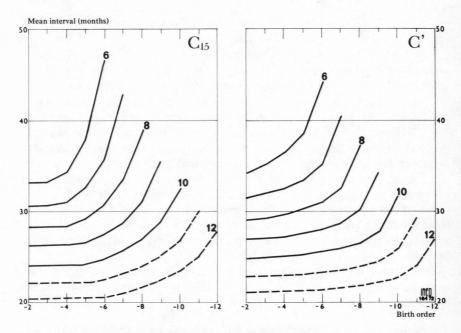

Fig. A.3.   Birth intervals, by birth order and final size of family: Assumptions C_{15} and C'.

In applying C_{15}, I have assumed that fecundability decreases over 15 years, as in B_{15}; intrauterine mortality is constant and equal to 25%; and the nonsusceptible periods have the distributions given above. These distributions will not be repeated, since they are common to the rest of the applications that follow.

The starting level of fecundability is higher than 0.50 (0.578) in order to partially compensate for the effect of intrauterine mortality.

The result (left side of fig. A.3) differs from the preceding ones in two ways: the curves are much farther apart ($I_6 - I_{10} = 9.1$ months, versus 5.3 and 3.5 previously); and the widening is somewhat smaller ($R_6 - R_{10} = 5.0$, versus 5.4 and 8.3).

The greater dispersion is a direct consequence of the introduction of two additional sources of variation: a distribution of nonsusceptible periods and intrauterine mortality. But on the whole the result still is not satisfactory.

Before abandoning it, let us compare it to the result of the next application C'.

In the C' model, I have exchanged the hypotheses: fecundability is constant (at 0.50 level); and intrauterine mortality increases with age, from 16% to 100% (such that effective fecundability reaches zero).

The result (fig. A.3, right side) is very close to C_{15}; it is even better on one point—the increase of the last intervals is almost independent of the final family size ($R_6 - R_{10} = 1.9$). We arrive, therefore, at the following double conclusion:

1. A continuous increase in intrauterine mortality can be used to explain the mean increase of the last intervals just as well as a decrease in fecundability.

2. The "fan effect" (in the increase of these intervals) is greatly reduced by the increase in intrauterine mortality.

We must note that in both cases, the choice of hypotheses must be such that effective fecundability always approaches zero. Otherwise, one obtains a design of the type C'' where we have assumed intrauterine mortality to reach a maximum of 50% instead of 100% (fig. A.4).

To improve the model, we have then assumed that both fecundability and intrauterine mortality were functions of age (fig. A.5).

In application C'_{15}, the hypothesis of model C_{15} is used for fecundability,

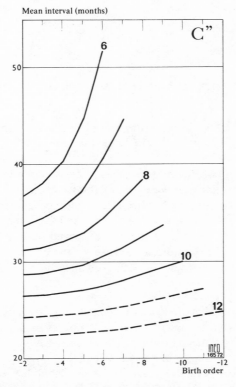

Fig. A.4. Birth intervals, by birth order and final size of family: Assumption C''.

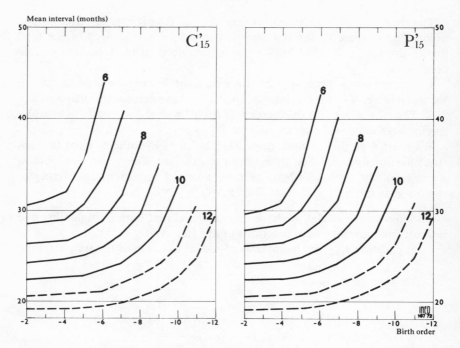

Fig. A.5. Birth intervals, by birth order and final size of family: Assumptions C'_{15} and P'_{15}.

and that of model C' for intrauterine mortality: the former decreases over a 15-year period, from 0.578 to 0; the latter increases continuously from 16% to 100%.

The result is excellent: the mean increase (R_m) is very close to the observed values (6.7 months), and the widening of the network is fairly small ($R_6 - R_{10} = 3.5$). Also, the network has been tightened up: $I_6 - I_{10} = 8.2$ months. All these figures are fairly close to those observed for Japan, or for historical France, as well as to estimates that may be derived from other observations. (Because of the fairly pronounced increase, in the case of historical France, between the [1–2] interval and the others, I have based the comparison on the [2–3] interval.)

We can thus consider that our principal objective has been attained. However, to show that the result obtained is not affected much by variations in the *level* of the parameters used, I have studied a hypothesis similar to the last one, in which starting fecundability is equal to 0.833 (or 0.45 in monthly values), which corresponds to an effective fecundability of 0.700 (or 0.33 monthly).

This hypothesis P'_{15} leads to a higher mean final family size (8.1) and to a slight tightening of both the fan ($R_6 - R_{10} = 3.2$) and the network ($I_6 - I_{10} = 7.3$). This still fits the data for historical France very well, except for the 1–2 interval, which is too short in this latter case.

Role of Distribution of Ages at Marriage and at Permanent Sterility

I shall start by taking sterility into account. Starting from the distribution given in chapter 6, we have assumed that women married at age 22.5 years could become sterile at 27.5, 32.5, 37.5, 42.5, or 45 years of age. Table A.3 shows the proportions belonging to these different groups and the lengths of their reproductive lives (in quarters). (It was unnecessary to consider the case of women already sterile at the time of marriage, since their final family size is obviously zero.)

To these cohorts, I have applied the hypotheses of model C_{15}, by stopping the process after 20, 40, 60 or 80 quarters (the C_{15} model itself corresponding to a reproductive period equal to 90 quarters). Then I have recombined the results for each final family size by a double weighting, one taking account of the proportion of families of a given size, for a specific length of reproductive life, the other taking account of the distribution of lengths of reproductive life (column 2 of table A.3).

What results is a network I shall call C_{15}^s (cf. fig. A.6, left). Compared with C_{15}', this network provides two reasons for dissatisfaction: (1) the increase of the last intervals is somewhat low (5.3 instead of 6.7 months); and (2),

Table A.3.   Duration of Fecund Life

Mean Age at Onset of Sterility	Number of Women (%)	Duration of Fecund Life (3-Month Unit)	Periods of Fecundity
Age at marriage: 22.5			
27.5	4	20	0 to 20
32.5	6	40	0 to 40
37.5	16	60	0 to 60
42.5	31	80	0 to 80
45.0	43	90	0 to 90
	100		
Age at marriage: 27.5			
32.5	7	20	20 to 40
37.5	17	40	20 to 60
42.5	32	60	20 to 80
45.0	44	70	20 to 90
	100		

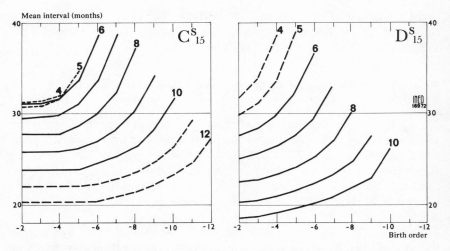

Fig. A.6. Birth intervals, by birth order and final size of family: Assumptions C_{15}^s and D_{15}^s.

more important, the curves for family sizes less than 7 (25% of all families) cross and intermingle.

This anomaly results because the group of small-sized families consists mainly of women who become sterile early, even before their fecundability begins to decline (remember that intrauterine mortality is constant in hypotheses C_{15}). The increase of the intervals has thus not had time to occur.

But this phenomenon is not found at all in the *observed* networks. In these, the mean final family size varies from 7.2 to 8.1: it is thus slightly higher than that resulting from my model (7.1), but I have eliminated families with fewer than 5 children from the observations. If we also exclude them from network C_{15}^s, the mean becomes 7.3, a value very close to that of Japan and Martinique. In these two samples, the families of 5 children show a final interval much longer than the next-to-last: my result is thus significantly different.

The result, in my opinion, is that it is not realistic to assume that the decrease in fecundability is strictly a function of the woman's age, with sterility coming at a given time to brutally interrupt a process of continuous decrease. Rather, we must admit that the onset of sterility is (almost always) preceded by a phase of decline in fecundity, no matter what the age at which sterility occurs (at least after some minimum age—30 or 35 years, for example). (One could attempt to verify this point by studying separately the women who had their last child before age 35.)

I have next made the assumption that all women marry at age 27.5 years, instead of 22.5 years, and then merge into the preceding cohorts at this age, with the same hypotheses (cf. table A.3). I have thus created four networks,

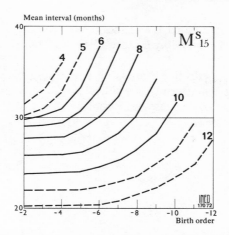

Fig. A.7. Birth intervals, by birth order and final size of family: Assumption M_{15}^s.

corresponding respectively to periods of fecundity covering quarters 20 to 40, 20 to 60, 20 to 80 and 20 to 90, with the distribution of women among the several cohorts calculated as before.

Again, these four networks can be combined into a single network, D_{15}^s. This network is not in itself of great interest; its mean final family size is 5.2, or 2 children fewer than for C_{15}^s. As a result, the network can almost be superimposed on C_{15}^s by a simple translation.

By recombining networks C_{15}^s and D_{15}^s, we introduce the last "distribution": that of age at marriage. It is reduced to two classes, each one requiring a large number of previous calculations.[1] I have assumed that 77% of the women married at 22.5 years and 23% at 27.5 years.

The resulting network (M_{15}^s, fig. A.7) is a great improvement over network C_{15}^s. This follows logically from the fact that, for example, the curve for a final family size of 5 is approximately an average of the one for a final family size of 6 in C_{15}^s and the one for a final family size of 4 in D_{15}^s.

We may note that the defects of network C_{15}^s (for small final family size) are reduced but not eliminated: my preceding conclusions thus stand. But we can say that taking age at marriage into account is, finally, of limited interest. In the matter of concern here, it is the changes in the parameters *at the end of the reproductive period* that are important.

My final conclusions will thus be the following:
1. The increase of intrauterine mortality with age, and the decrease of fecundability at the end of the reproductive period, play a symmetrical role.

1. When this work was done, I had access to only a very small computer.

But it is necessary that either the former tends to 100% or the latter tends to zero (i.e., effective fecundability must reach zero at the end of the reproductive life).

2. The decrease of effective fecundability must take place whatever the age at onset of permanent sterility. In other words, permanent sterility must occur after a period of decrease in fecundity.

Appendix B
Tables

Table B.1. Mean Live-Birth Intervals (in Months), by Birth Order and Final Family Size (Japan, Rural Families)

Total Number of Live Births	Birth Orders											
	0-1[a]	1-2	2-3	3-4	4-5	5-6	6-7	7-8	8-9	9-10	10-11	11-12
5	28.6	40.0	40.4	43.4	50.8							
6	25.1	35.1	37.1	37.8	39.2	46.9						
7	23.5	32.9	33.2	34.2	34.6	36.9	43.6					
8	21.3	30.7	31.2	32.1	32.4	32.7	35.1	41.2				
9	20.6	28.7	29.6	30.7	29.4	30.8	30.6	33.2	40.5			
10	20.4	26.3	29.4	28.1	27.1	28.5	28.2	28.5	34.6	34.3		
11	20.2	26.2	25.5	25.7	25.8	25.9	26.4	26.5	25.6	29.0	34.6	
12	19.0	26.8	25.5	26.4	25.7	25.7	24.1	24.8	23.7	24.8	28.7	31.2
8 and more (mean: 9.0)	20.8	28.9	29.6	30.4	29.9	30.6						
Last intervals[b]					$-(n-4)$	$-(n-3)$	$-(n-2)$	$-(n-1)$	$-(n)$			
					29.9	30.4	30.5	33.5	39.2			

SOURCE: Okasaki 1951 (ref. 351), table X.

[a] Interval between marriage and first birth.

[b] n = order of last birth within each family.

Table B.2. Mean Live-Birth Intervals (in Months), by Birth Order and Final Family Size (France, Eighteenth Century)

Total Number of Live Births	Number of Families	0–1 [a]	1–2	2–3	3–4	4–5	5–6	6–7	7–8	8–9	9–10	10–11	11–12
5	61	13.6	24.6	28.5	32.9	39.8							
6	76	15.1	24.9	28.5	31.8	32.6	39.9						
7	60	15.6	22.2	26.9	27.1	28.8	33.0	39.2					
8	80	12.6	22.8	25.6	25.4	27.3	28.4	30.3	37.2				
9	52	12.7	20.9	24.2	23.4	26.1	25.9	26.3	30.6	38.1			
10	41	14.1	20.1	22.5	24.6	25.4	22.4	24.6	24.8	29.2	34.9		
11	36	11.6	19.5	21.8	21.4	22.8	25.0	24.1	24.7	24.3	29.4	30.4	
12	20	10.7	18.3	20.8	20.9	23.9	22.7	19.7	20.7	20.7	26.1	25.0	28.9
13 and more (mean: 13.7)	24	11.0	16.1	17.7	19.6	18.7	20.0	19.0	18.5	22.8	20.9	22.5	22.9

Birth Orders

Last intervals [b]

	$n-6$ / $-n-5$	$n-5$ / $-n-4$	$n-4$ / $-n-3$	$n-3$ / $-n-2$	$n-2$ / $-n-1$	$n-1$ / $-n$
Total 450	20.5	20.7	23.2	22.1	22.5	31.4

SOURCE: Leridon 1967 (ref. 029), table 1.
[a] Interval between marriage and first birth.
[b] n = order of last birth within each family.

Table B.3. Characteristic Values of Various Networks of Birth Intervals (Live-Birth Intervals in Families of Size 8 or Over)

Sample	Mean Family Size	Number of Families	Interval Order[b]										
			1–2	–3	–4	–5	–6	–7	–8	–9	–10	–11	–12
France (18th century)	9.8	253	20.5	23.1	23.4	25.0	25.2						
						24.1	24.1						
Japan	9.0	ca. 1,300	28.9	29.6	30.4	29.9	30.6	25.3	26.0	28.9	34.8		
						29.9	30.4						
Martinique	9.8	87	25.2	23.1	24.7	24.4	25.8	23.6	26.4	26.6	31.3		
							24.1						
Hutterites	11.6	155	19.9	20.5	21.6	22.2	22.7	23.7	23.7	23.6	24.9	27.2	30.3
								22.5					
Amish	10.0	266	20.5	21.2	22.1	23.2	24.8	25.0	26.8	28.8	34.1		
								23.7					
France (1954)	8[a]	360	21.6	24.0	26.4	27.6	31.0	33.6	42.7				

SOURCES: France (18th century): Leridon 1967, (ref. 029).
Japan: Okasaki 1951 (ref. 351).
Martinique: personal data.
Hutterites: From Sheps 1965 (ref. 353).
Amish: Cross and McKusick 1970 (ref. 324).
France (1954): INSEE, unpublished data.
[a] Families of size 8 only.
[b] On second line, intervals are computed backward from the last birth in each family.

Table B.4. Data for Model SIMNAT: Distribution of 1,000 Pregnancies by Duration of Nonsusceptible Period (Including Gestation)

Duration in Months	Live Birth No Breast-feeding	Short NSP[a]	Long NSP	Fetal Death Duration in Months	
6	0	0	0	1	40
7	0	5	0	2	70
8	0	5	0	3	120
9	0	5	0	4	170
10	100	60	50	5	200
11	400	210	70	6	170
12	300	165	30	7	120
13	140	90	25	8	70
14	60	50	15	9	30
15	0	20	20	10	10
16	—	25	20		
17	—	30	20	Mean	5.0
18	—	30	30		
19	—	35	40		
20	—	40	50		
21	—	35	60		
22	—	30	65		
23	—	30	70		
24	—	25	65		
25	—	20	60		
26	—	20	55		
27	—	20	50		
28	—	15	45		
29	—	15	40		
30	—	10	35		
31	—	5	30		
32	—	5	25		
33	—	0	30		
Mean	11.7	15.8	21.8		

Nonsusceptible period.

Table B.5. Data for Model SIMNAT: Distributions of First Marriages by Age of Woman (for 1,000 Women Aged 15 Years and Over)

Age in Years	Early Marriage	Late Marriage
15	100	14
16	162	19
17	177	27
18	168	34
19	130	44
20	89	54
21	61	63
22	41	71
23	26	78
24	16	83
25	11	77
26	7	67
27	4	58
28	3	48
29	2	40
30	1	32
31	1	24
32	—	18
33	—	13
34	—	11
35	—	9
36	—	8
37	—	7
38	—	6
39	—	5
40	—	4
41	—	4
42	—	2
43	—	2
44	—	1
Mean age	18.8	25.2

Table B.6. Data for Model SIMNAT: Distribution of 10,000 Women by Age at Onset of Permanent Sterility

Age in Years	Low sterility	Medium Sterility	High Sterility
Under 15	0	300	300
15	60	60	60
16	60	60	60
17	60	60	60
18	60	60	60
19	60	60	60
20	60	72	72
21	60	72	72
22	60	84	84
23	60	84	84
24	60	84	84
25	72	100	108
26	72	100	108
27	84	110	120
28	84	114	132
29	84	120	132
30	108	130	156
31	108	150	204
32	120	190	276
33	132	260	372
34	132	330	492
35	156	400	624
36	204	500	732
37	276	550	840
38	372	600	936
39	492	650	768
40	624	700	624
41	732	700	552
42	840	700	480
43	936	600	408
44	768	500	336
45	624	400	264
46	552	320	192
47	480	280	120
48	408	200	24
49	336	150	4
50	264	120	0
51	192	30	0
52	120	0	0
53	24	0	0
54	4	0	0
Mean age	41.0	37.7	36.0

Table B.7. Data for Model SIMNAT: Risk of Intrauterine Mortality by Age of Mother

Age in Years	Rate per 1,000	Age in Years	Rate per 1,000
15	118	33	163
16	118	34	170
17	118	35	177
18	118	36	185
19	118	37	194
20	119	38	205
21	120	39	217
22	122	40	228
23	123	41	242
24	125	42	259
25	127	43	280
26	130	44	300
27	134	45	320
28	137	46	340
29	142	47	360
30	146	48	380
31	157	49	400
32	152		

Classified Bibliography

0 Methods of Measurement

0.0 General Works
0.1 Usual Fertility Indexes
0.2 Reproduction
0.3 Birth Intervals

1 Natural Fertility

1.0 Physiology of Reproduction
1.00 *General Works*
1.01 *Puberty*
1.02 *Menopause*
1.03 *Ovulatory Cycle*
1.04 *Duration of Pregnancy— Prematurity*
1.1 Factors
1.10 *General Studies*
1.11 *Fecundability— Frequency of Intercourse*
1.12 *Intrauterine Mortality*
1.120 Demographic Aspects
1.121 Etiology
1.122 Perinatal Mortality
1.13 *Postpartum Sterility— Breast-feeding*
1.14 *Permanent and Temporary Sterility*
1.2 Characteristics of Births
1.21 *Sex*
1.22 *Multiple Births*
1.23 *Anomalies*
1.4 Models
1.5 Data on Natural Fertility

2 The Control of Fertility

2.2 Methods (Contraception, Abortion, Sterilization)
2.20 *General Studies*
2.22 *Rhythm (Calendar and Temperature)*
2.24 *Oral Contraceptives*
2.25 *Intrauterine Devices*
2.28 *Abortion*
2.29 *Sterilization*
2.3 Measurement of Effectiveness
2.31 *Effectiveness: Individual Level*
2.32 *Demographic Effectiveness*
2.4 Models (See 1.4)

171

0 Methods of Measurement

0.0   General Works

000 Barclay, G. W. 1958. *Techniques of population analysis*. New York:
      John Wiley.
001 Cox, P. R. 1970. *Demography*. Cambridge: Cambridge University Press.
002 Hajnal, J. 1959. The study of fertility and reproduction: A survey of
      thirty years. In *Thirty years research in human fertility: Retrospect
      and prospect*. New York: Milbank Memorial Fund Quarterly.
003 Henry L. 1972. *Démographie: Analyse et modèles*. Paris: Larousse.
004 Henry, L. 1972. *On the measurement of human fertility: Selected
      writings*. Amsterdam: Elsevier.
005 Keyfitz, N., and Flieger, W. 1971. *Population: Facts and methods of
      demography*. San Francisco: Freeman.
006 United Nations. 1967. *Manual IV. Methods of estimating basic
      demographic measures from incomplete data*. New York: United
      Nations Population Studies, no. 42.
007 Pressat, R. 1969. *L'analyse démographique*. 2d ed. Paris: P.U.F.
008 Pressat, R. 1972. *Demographic analysis*. Chicago: Aldine-Atherton.
009 Ryder, N. B. 1959. Fertility. In *The study of population*, ed. P. M.
      Hauser and O. D. Duncan. Chicago: University of Chicago Press.
010 Shyrock, H. S.; Siegel, J. S.; et al. 1971. *The Methods and materials
      of demography*. Washington, D.C.: U.S. Bureau of the Census.

0.1   Usual Fertility Indexes

011 Bourgeois-Pichat, J. 1950. *Mesure de la fécondité des populations*.
      Travaux et Documents, no. 12. Paris: I.N.E.D.–P.U.F.
012 Bumpass, L., and Westoff, C. F. 1969. The prediction of completed
      fertility. *Demography* 6 (4):445–54.
013 Coale, A. J., and Trussell, L. 1974. Model fertility schedules. *Pop.
      Index* 40:185–258.
014 Henry, L. 1953. Fécondité des mariages: Nouvelle méthode de
      mesure. Travaux et Documents, no. 16. Paris: I.N.E.D.–P.U.F.
015 Henry, L. 1953. Fondements théoriques des mesures de la fécondité
      naturelle. *Revue de l'Institut Intern. de Stat.* 21(3):135–51.
016 Wunsch, G. 1966. Courbes de Gompertz et perspectives de fécondité.
      Recherches Econ. de Louvain, no. 6.
017 Wunsch, G. 1967. Les mesures de la natalité: Quelques applications
      à la Belgique. *Fac. Sc. Econ. Polit.*, Louvain, n.s., no. 28.

0.2   Reproduction

018 Henry, L. 1965. Réflexions sur les taux de reproduction (with a
      comment by J. Bourgeois-Pichat). *Population* 20(1):53–76.

019 Keyfitz, N. 1968. *Introduction to the mathematics of population.* Reading, Mass.: Addison–Wesley.

020 Lotka, A. 1934. Théorie analytique des associations biologiques. Vol. 2. Paris: Herman.

021 Stolnitz, G. J., Ryder, N. B. 1956. Recent discussion of the net reproduction rate. In *Demographic analysis: Selected readings,* ed. J. J. Spengler and O. D. Duncan. Glencoe, Ill.: Free Press.

022 Wunsch, G. 1967. Les mesures de la natalité: Quelque applications à la Belgique. *Fac. Sc. Econ. Polit.,* Louvain, n.s. no. 28.

0.3 Birth Intervals

023 Cantrelle, P., Leridon, H. 1971. Breast-feeding, mortality in childhood and fertility in a rural zone of Senegal. *Pop. Studies,* 25 (3):505–533.

024 Chen, L. C.; Ahmed, S.; Gesche, M.; and Mosley, W. H. 1974. A prospective study of birth interval dynamics in rural Bangladesh. *Pop. Studies* 28(2):277–97.

025 Dandekar, K. 1963. Analysis of birth intervals of a set of Indian women. *Eugenics Quart.* 10(2):73–78.

026 Dandekar, K. 1959. Intervals between confinements. *Eugenics Quart.* 6(3):180–186.

027a D'Souza, S. 1973. Interlive-birth intervals of non-contraceptive populations: A data analytic study. *Social Action* 23:404–25.

027b D'Souza, S. 1974. *Closed birth intervals: A data analytic study.* New Delhi: Sterling Publ. Pvt. Ltd.

028 Henry, L. 1958. Intervals between confinements in the absence of birth control. *Eugenics Quart.* 5(4):200–211.

029 Leridon, H. 1967. Les intervalles entre naissances: Nouvelles données d'observation. *Population* 22(5):821–40.

030 Poole, W. K. 1973. Fertility measures based on birth interval data. *Theor. Pop. Biol.* 4(3):357–87.

031 Potter, R. G. 1963. Birth intervals: Structure and change. *Pop. Studies* 17:155–66.

032 Potter, R. G.; Wyon, J. B.; Parker, M.; and Gordon, J. E. 1965. A case study of birth interval dynamics. *Pop. Studies* 19(1):81–96.

033 Sagi, P. C. 1959. A component analysis of birth intervals among two-child white couples. In *Thirty years of research in human fertility: Retrospect and prospect,* part II. New York, Milbank Memorial Fund Quarterly.

034 Sheps, M. C.; Menken, J. A.; Ridley, J. C.; and Lingner, J. W. 1970. Truncation effect in closed and open birth interval data. *J. Am. Stat. Ass.* 65:678–93.

035 Sheps, M. C., and Menken, J. A. 1972. Distribution of birth intervals according to the sampling frame. *Theor. Pop. Biol.* 3(1):1–26.

036 Sheps, M. C., and Perrin, E. B. 1964. The distribution of birth intervals under a class of stochastic fertility models. *Pop. Studies* 17:321–31.

037 Srinivasan, K. 1967. A probability model applicable to the study of inter-live birth intervals and random segments of the same. *Pop. Studies* 21(1):63–70. (See comment by H. Leridon in *Pop. Studies* 23 [March 1969]:101–4.)

038 Srinivasan, K. 1970. Findings and implications of a correlation analysis of the closed and the open birth intervals. *Demography* 7(4):401–10.

039 Wolfers, D. 1968. Determinants of birth intervals and their means. *Pop. Studies* 22(2):253–62.

1 Natural Fertility

1.0 Physiology of Reproduction

1.00 General Works

040a *Biological components of human reproduction.* 1969. Technical Reports Series, no. 435. Geneva: WHO.

040b Frisch, R. E. 1975. Demographic implications of the biological determinants of female fecundity. *Soc. Biol.* 22(1):17–22.

041 Gautray, J. P. 1968. *Reproduction humaine.* Paris: Masson.

042 Hervet, E., and Barrat, J. 1968. *Stérilité, contraception.* Paris: J. B. Baillière et Fils.

043 Loraine, J. A., and Bell, E. T. 1968. *Fertility and contraception in the human female.* Edinburgh and London: E. and S. Livingstone.

044 Odell, W., and Moyer, D. 1971. *Physiology of reproduction.* Saint Louis: Mosby Publishers.

045 Page, E. W.; Villee, C. A.; and Villee, D. B. 1972. Human reproduction. Philadelphia: W. B. Saunders.

046 Parkes, A. S. 1973. The social impact of human reproduction (lecture). *J. Biosoc. Sci.* 5(2):195–204.

047 *Reproductive biology.* 1968. Proceedings of the first seminar, 26–28 March, 1966, New Delhi, sponsored by Central Family Planning Institute and Indian Council of Medical Research. New Delhi.

048 Udry, J. R., et al. 1971. Pregnancy testing as a fertility measurement technique: A preliminary report on field results. *Am. J. Public Health* 61(2):344–52.

049 Vincent, P. 1956. Données biométriques sur la conception et la grossesse. *Population* 11(1):1–29.

1.01 Puberty

050 Frisch, R. E., and Revelle, R. 1971. Height and weight at menarche and a hypothesis of menarche. *Arch. Dis. Childhood* 46(249):695–701.

051 MacMahon, B. 1973. Age at menarche, United States. NCHS Vital

and Health Statistics, series 11, no. 133. Washington, D.C.: U.S. Dept. HEW.

052 Montagu, M. F. A. 1946. Adolescent sterility. Springfield, Ill.: Charles C. Thomas.

053 Tanner, J. M. 1968. Earlier maturation in man. *Sci. Am.* 218(1):26.

054 Tanner, J. M. 1973. Trend toward earlier menarche in London, Oslo, Copenhagen, the Netherlands and Hungary. Nature 243: 95–96.

055 Weir, J., et al. 1971. Race and age at menarche. *Am. J. Obstet. Gynecol.* 111:594–96.

1.02 Menopause

056 Bourliere, F.; Cendron, M.; and Clement, F. 1966. Le vieillissement individuel dans une population rurale française: Etude de la commune de Plozévet. *Bull. Mém. Soc. Anthrop. Paris,* ser. 11, 10:41–101.

057 Bourliere, F.; Clement, F.; and Parot, S. 1966. Normes de vieillissement morphologique et physiologique d'une population de niveau socio-économique élevé de la région parisienne. *Bull. Mém. Soc. Anthrop. Paris,* ser. 11, 10:11–39.

058 McKinlay, S.; Jefferys, M.; and Thompson, B. 1972. An investigation of the age at menopause. *J. Biosoc. Sci.* 4(2):161–73.

059 McKinlay, S. and McKinlay, J. 1973. Selected studies of the menopause (annotated bibliography). *J. Biosoc. Sci.* 5(4):533–55.

060 MacMahon, B., and Worcester, J. 1966. *Age at menopause: United States, 1960–62.* Series 11, no. 19. Washington, D.C.: National Center for Health Statistics.

061 Tisserand-Perrier, M., and Bourliere, F. 1953. Quelques caractéristiques de deux populations de femmes âgées parisiennes. *Biotypologie* 14 (3–4):95–111.

062 Tisserand-Perrier, M., and Bourliere, F. 1953. Recherches sur la ménopause. *Gynecol. Obst.* 52(1):43–56.

063 Wyon, J. B.; Finner, S. L.; and Gordon, J. E. 1966. Differential age at menopause in the rural Punjab, India. *Pop. Index* 32(3):328.

1.03 Ovulatory Cycle

064 Collett, M. E., et al. 1954. The effect of age upon the pattern of the menstrual cycle. *Fertil. Steril.* 5:437.

065 Farris, E. J. 1952. A formula for selecting the optimum time for conception. *Am. J. Obst. Gynecol.* 63:1143–46.

066a Farris, E. J. 1956. Human ovulation and fertility. Philadelphia: J. B. Lippincott.

066b Frisch, R. E., and McArthur, J. W. 1974. Menstrual cycles: Fatness as a determinant of minimum weight for height necessary for their maintenance or onset. *Science* 185:949–51.

067a Matsumoto, S. 1964. Statistical survey of the length of the menstrual cycle and the duration of menstruation in 3000 ovulatory cycles based upon BBT findings. 7th IPPF Conference (Singapore). *Excerpta Medica*, I.C.S. no. 72, pp. 202–5.

067*b* Treolar, A. E.; Boynton, R. E.; Behn, B. G.; and Brown, B. W. 1967. Variation of the human menstrual cycle through reproductive life. *Intern. J. Fertil.* 12(1, part 2):77–126.

068 Vincent, P. 1957. Statistiques relatives à l'ovulation, à la menstruation et à la grossesse. Rio de Janeiro, *Bull. I.S.S.* 35(2):1–16.

069 Vollmann, R. F. 1953. Die Lange des Prämentruum in Regression zum Alter der Frau. *Gynaecologia* 135(2):78–83.

070 Vollmann, R. F. 1952–53. Uber Fertilität und Sterilität der Frau innerhalb des Menstruations cyclus. *Archiv. Gynaekol.* 182:602–22.

1.04 Duration of Pregnancy—Prematurity

071 Chase, H. C., and Byrnes, M. E. 1972. Trends in prematurity: United States, 1950–67. Washington, D.C.: U.S. Center for Health Statistics, Vital and Health Statistics, series 3, Analytical Stud., no. 1. (Jan.).

072 Gibson, J. R., and McKeown, T. 1950. Observation on all births (23,970) in Birmingham, 1947. I: Duration of gestation. *British J. Soc. Med.* 4:221–33.

073*a* Hammes, L. M., and Trolar, A. E. 1970. Gestational interval from vital records. *Amer. J. Public Health* 60(8):1496–1505.

073*b* Leridon, H. 1974. Etude de la clientèle et du champ d'attraction d'un service hospitalier. *Population* 29(2):291–312.

1.1 Factors

1.10 General Studies

074 Bourgeois-Pichat, J. 1965. Les facteurs de la fécondité non dirigée. *Population* 20(3):383–424.

075 Bourgeois-Pichat, J. 1954. La mesure de la fécondité des populations humaines. *Proc. World Pop. Confer.* (*Rome*) 4:249–61.

076 Bourgeois-Pichat, J. 1967. Social and biological determinants of human fertility in nonindustrial societies. *Proc. Am. Philos. Soc.* 3(3):160–63.

077 Henry, L. 1963. Aspects biologiques de la fécondité. *Proc. Roy. Soc.*, ser. B, 159:81–93.

078 Henry, L. 1965. French statistical research in natural fertility. In *Public Health and population change*, ed. M. C. Sheps and J. C. Ridley, pp. 333–50. Pittsburgh: University of Pittsburgh Press.

079 Henry, L. 1961. La fécondité naturelle: Observation, théorie, résultats. *Population* 16(4):625–36.

080 Leridon, H. 1967. Les intervalles entre naissances: Nouvelles données d'observation. *Population* 22(5):821–40.

081 Leridon, H. 1973. Natalité, saisons et conjoncture économique. Travaux et Documents, no. 66, Paris: I.N.E.D.–P.U.F.

082 Nag, M. 1962. Factors affecting human fertility in non-industrial societies: A cross-cultural study. *Yale University Publications in Anthropology.* New Haven: Yale University.

083 Pearl, R. 1939. The natural history of the population. New York: Oxford University Press.

084 Potter, R. G. 1963. Birth intervals: Structure and change. *Pop. Studies* 17:155–62.

085 Potter, R. G.; Gordon, J.; Parker, M.; Wyon, J. 1965. A case study of birth intervals dynamics. *Pop. Studies* 19(1):81–96.

086 Potter, R. G.; New, M.; Wyon, J.; and Gordon, J. 1965. Applications of field studies to research on the physiology of human reproduction. *J. Chronic Diseases* 18:1125–40.

087 Stone, A. 1955. *Biological factors influencing human fertility.* Vol. 1. Congrès mondial de la population, Rome, 1954, New York: O.N.U.

088 Vincent, P. 1961 Recherches sur la fécondité biologique. Travaux et Documents, no. 37. Paris: I.N.E.D.–P.U.F.

1.11 Fecundability–Frequency of Intercourse

089 Barrett, J. C. 1970. An analysis of coital patterns. *J. Biosoc. Sci.* 2(4): 351–357.

090 Barrett, J. C. 1971. Fecundability and coital frequency. *Pop. Studies* 25(2):309–13.

091 Barrett, J. C., and Marshall, J. 1969. The risk of conception on different days of the menstrual cycle. *Pop. Studies* 23(3):455–61.

092 Berquo, E. S., et al. 1968. Levels and variations in fertility in São Paulo. *Milbank Mem. Fund Quart.* 46(3), part 2:167–85.

093 Bongaarts, J. 1975. A method for the estimation of fecundability. *Demography* 12(4):645–60.

094 Gini, C. 1926. Decline in the birth-rate and "fecundability" of women. *Eugenics Rev.,* January.

095 Gini, C. 1924. Premières recherches sur la fécondabilité de la femme. *Proc. Math. Congr.* Toronto, pp. 889–92.

096 Glasser, J. H., and Lachenbruch, P. A. 1968. Observations on the relationship between frequency and timing of intercourse and the probability of conception. *Pop. Studies* 22(3):399–407.

097 Halbert, D. R. 1971. Anovulation following use of oral contraceptives: A review. *North Carolina Med. J.* 32:379–83.

098 Henry, L. 1964. Mortalité intra-utérine et fécondabilité. *Population* 19(5):899–940.

100 Jain, A. K. 1969. Fecundability and its relation to age in a sample of Taiwanese women. *Pop. Studies* 23(1):69–85.

101 Jain, A. K. 1969. Relative fecundability of users and non-users of contraception. *Soc. Biol.* 16(1):39–43.

102 Jain, A. K. 1969. Socio-economic correlates of fecundability in a sample of Taiwanese women. *Demography* 6(1):75–90.

103 James, W. H. 1971. The distribution of coitus within the human intermenstruum. *J. Biosoc. Sci.* 3(2):159–71.

104 James, W. H. 1963. Estimates of fecundability. *Pop. Studies* 17(1): 57–65. (See comment by L. Henry in *Pop. Studies* 18[2]:175–180.)

105 James, W. H. 1965. Parameters of the menstrual cycle, and the efficiency of rhythm methods of contraception. *Pop. Studies* 19(1):45–64. (See comment by R. G. Potter in *Pop. Studies* 20[2]:223–32.)

106 James, W. H. 1968. The mathematics of the menstrual cycle. *Pop. Studies* 22(3):409–13.

107 Kinsey, A. C.; Pomeroy, W. B.; and Martin, C. E. 1948. Sexual behavior in the human male. Philadelphia: Saunders.

108 Kinsey, A. C.; Pomeroy, W. B.; Martin, C. E.; and Gebhard, P. H. 1953. *Sexual behavior in the human female*. Philadelphia: Saunders.

109 Lachenbruch, P. A. 1967. Frequency and timing of intercourse: Its relation to the probability of conception. *Pop. Studies* 21(1):23–31.

110a Majumdar, H., and Sheps, M. C. 1970. Estimations of a type I geometric distribution from observations on conception times. *Demography* 7(3):349–60.

110b Menken, J. A. 1975. Estimating fecundability. Ph.D. diss., Princeton University.

111 Mustafa, A. F. M. 1973. Approaches to the measurement of fecundability: An analytical review. *Egypt. Pop. Fam. Plan Rev.* 6(2):131–44.

112 Olusanaya, P. O. 1971. The problem of multiple causation in population analysis, with particular reference to the polygamy-fertility hypothesis. *Sociol. Rev.* 19(2):165–78.

113 Potter, R. G. 1961. Length of the fertile period. *Milbank Mem. Fund Quart.* 39(1):132–62.

114 Potter, R. G., and Parker, M. P. 1964. Predicting the time required to conceive. *Pop. Studies* 18(1):99–116.

115 Potter, R. G.; Sagi, P.; and Westoff, C. F. 1962. Knowledge of the ovulatory cycle and coital frequency as factors affecting conception and contraception. *Milbank Mem. Fund Quart* 40(1):46–58.

116 Potter, R. G.; Sakoda, J. M.; and Feinberg, W. E. 1968. Variable fecundability and the timing of births. *Eugenics Quart* 15(3):155–63.

117 Potter, R. G.; Westoff, C. F.; and Sagi, P. 1963. Delays in conception: A discrepancy re-examined. *Eugenics Quart.* 10(2):53–58.

118 Sheps, M. C. 1964. On the time required for conception. *Pop. Studies* 18(1):85–96.

119 Simon, P.; Gondonneau, J.; Mironer, L.; and Dourlen-Rollier, A. M. 1972. Rapport sur le comportement sexuel des Français. Paris: Julliard et Charron.

120 Singh, S. N., and Bhaduri, T. 1972. Maximum likelihood estimations for the parameters of a continuous time model for first conception. *Demography* 9(4):249–56.

121 Tietze, C. 1968. Fertility after discontinuation of intrauterine and hormonal contraception. *Int. J. Fertil.* 13(4):385–89.

122 Tietze, C. 1960. Probability of pregnancy resulting from a single unprotected coitus. *Fertil. Steril.* 11:484–88.

123 Tietze, C. 1956. Statistical contributions to the study of human fertility. *Fertil. Steril.* 7(1):88–94.

124 Tietze, C. Guttmacher, A. F.; and Rubin, S. 1950. Time required for conception in 1727 planned pregnancies. *Fertil. Steril.* 1(4):338–46.

125 Vincent, P. 1956. Données biométriques sur la conception et la grossesse. *Population* 11(1):59–82.

126 Westoff, C. F. 1974. Coital frequency and contraception. *F. P. Perspectives* 6(3):136–41.

1.12 Intrauterine Mortality

1.120 Demographic Aspects

127 Abramson, F. D. 1973. Spontaneous fetal death in man. *Soc. Biol.* 20(4):375–403.

128 Abramson, F. D. 1971. Spontaneous fetal death in man: A methodological and analytical evaluation. Ph.D. diss. University of Michigan.

129 Bierman, J. M., et al. 1965. Analysis of the outcome of all pregnancies in a Community (Kauai). *Am. J. Obstet. Gynecol.* 91:37–45.

130 Coombs, L.; Freedman, R., and Namboothiri, D. N. 1969. Inferences about abortion from foetal mortality data. *Pop. Studies* 23(2):247–265.

131 Erhadt, C. L. 1963. Pregnancy losses in New York City, 1960. *Am. J. Public Health* 53(9):1337–52.

132 Freedman, R.; Coombs, L. C.; and Friedman, J. 1966. Social correlates of fetal mortality. *Milbank Mem. Fund Quart.* 44(3):327–44.

133 French, F. E., and Bierman, J. E. 1962. Probabilities of fetal mortality. *Public Health Rep.* 77(10):835–47.

134 Henry, L. 1964. Mortalité intra-utérine et fécondabilité. *Population* 19(5):899–940.

135 Jain, A. K. 1969. Pregnancy outcome and the time required for next conception. *Pop. Studies* 23(3):421–33.

136 Jain, A. K. 1969. Fetal wastage in a sample of Taiwanese women. *Milbank Mem. Fund Quart.*, 47(3, part 1):297–306.

137 James, W. H. 1963. Notes toward an epidemiology of spontaneous abortion. *Amer. J. Human Genet.* 15:223–40.

138 James, W. H. 1961. On the possibility of segregation in the propensity to spontaneous abortion in the human female. *Ann. Human Genet.* 25:207–13.

139 James, W. H. 1974. Spontaneous abortion and birth control. *J. Biosoc. Sci.* 6(1):23–41.

140 James, W. H. 1970. The incidence of spontaneous abortion. *Pop. Studies* 24(2):241–45.

141 Leridon, H. 1973. Démographie des échecs de la reproduction. In

Chromosomal errors in relation to reproductive failure, ed. A. Boué and C. Thibault, pp. 13–27. Paris: I.N.S.E.R.M.

142 Leridon, H. 1976. Facts and artifacts in the study of intra-uterine mortality: A reconsideration from pregnancy histories. *Pop. Studies* 30(2):319–36.

143 Mellin, G. W. 1962. Fetal life tables: A means of establishing perinatal rates of risk. *JAMA*, 180(1):11–14.

144a Naylor, A. F. 1974. Sequential aspects of spontaneous abortion: Maternal age, parity and pregnancy compensation artifact. *Soc. Biol.* 21(2):195–204.

144b Niswander, K. R., and Gordon, M. 1972. The women and their pregnancies. Philadelphia: W. B. Saunders.

145 Pettersson, F. 1968. *Epidemiology of early pregnancy wastage: Biological and social correlates of abortion. An investigation based on materials collected within Uppsala County, Sweden.* Stockholm: Svenska Bokforlaget.

146 Potter, R. G.; Wyon, J. B.; New, M.; and Gordon, J. E. 1965. Fetal wastage in eleven Punjab villages. *Human Biol.* 37:262–73.

147 *Rapport de statistiques sanitaires mondiales.* 1970. Vol. 23, no. 6. Sujet spécial: Mortalité foetale, 1945–67. Geneva: WHO.

148 Resseguie, L. J. 1974. Pregnancy wastage and age of mother among the Amish. *Human Biol.* 46(4):633–39.

149 Roth, D. B. 1963. The frequency of spontaneous abortion. *Int. J. Fertil.* 8(1):431–34.

150 Shapiro, S., and Abramowicz, M. 1969. Pregnancy outcome correlates identified through medical record-based information. *Am. J. Public Health* 59(9):1629–50.

151 Shapiro, S.; Jones, E.; and Densen, P. 1962. A life table of pregnancy terminations and correlates of fetal loss. *Milbank Mem. Fund Quart.* 40(1):7–45.

152 Shapiro, S.; Levine, H. S.; and Abramowicz, M. 1970. Factors associated with early and late fetal loss. *Adv. Planned Parenthood* 6:45–63.

153 *Spontaneous and induced abortion: Report of a WHO scientific group.* 1970. Technical report, series 461. Geneva: WHO.

154 Stevenson, A. C.; Warnock, H. A.; Dudgeon, M. Y.; and McClure, H. J. 1958. Observations on the results of pregnancies in women resident in Belfast (3 articles). *Ann. Human. Genet.* 23(4):382–420.

155 Stickle, G. 1968. Defective development and reproductive wastage in the United States. *Am. J. Obstet. Gynecol.* 100(3):442–47.

156 Taussig, F. J. 1936. Abortion, spontaneous and induced. Saint Louis: Mosby Co.

157 Taylor, W. F. 1964. On the methodology of measuring the probability of fetal death in a prospective study. *Human Biol.* 36(2):86–103.

158 Taylor, W. F. 1970. The probability of fetal death. In *Congenital malformations*, ed. F. C. Fraser and V. A. McKusick, pp. 307–20. Amsterdam and New York: Excerpta Medica.

159 Tietze, C., and Martin, C. E. 1957. Foetal deaths, spontaneous and

induced, in the urban white population of the United States. *Pop. Studies* 11(2):170–76.

160 Warburton, D., and Fraser, F. C. 1964. Spontaneous abortion risks in man: Data from reproductive histories collected in a medical genetics unit. *Am. J. Human Genet.* 16(1):1–25.

161 Weir, W. C., and Hendricks, C. H. 1969. The reproductive capacity of an infertile population. *Fertil. Steril.* 20(9):289–98.

162 Yerushalmy, J. et al. 1956. Longitudinal studies of pregnancy on the island of Kauai. Analysis of previous reproductive history. *Am. J. Obstet. Gynecol.* 71:80–96.

1.121 Etiology

163 Boué, J., and Boué, A. 1973. Anomalies chromosomiques dans les avortements spontanés. In *Chromosomal errors in relation to reproductive failure*, ed. A. Boué and C. Thibault, pp. 29–56. Paris: I.N.S.E.R.M.

164 Boué, J., and Boué, A. 1973. Chromosomal analysis of two consecutive abortuses in each of 43 women. *Human Genet.* 19:275–80.

165 Boué, J., and Boué, A. 1969. Fréquence des aberrations chromosomiques dans les avortements spontanés humains. *C. R. Acad. Sci.*, ser. D, 269:283–88.

166 Boué, J.; Boué, A.; and Lazar, P. 1967. Aberrations chromosomiques dans les avortements. *Annales genet.* 10(4):179–87.

167 Boué, J., and Lazar, P. 1969. Corrélation entre les différentes anomalies chromosomiques observées dans les avortements spontanés et les âges maternels. *C. R. Acad. Sci.* ser. D, 269:680–82.

168 Boué, J.; Philippe, E.; and Boué, A. 1969. Durée de la gestation et durée du développement dans les avortements humains dus à une anomalie chromosomique. *C. R. Acad. Sci.*, Ser. D, 269:420–23.

169 Bresler, J. B. 1970. Outcrossings in Caucasians and fetal loss. *Soc. Biol.* 17(1):17–25.

170 Carr, D. H. 1971. Chromosome and abortion. In *Advances in human genetics*, vol. 2, ed. Harry Harris and Kurt Huschhorn, pp. 201–57. New York: Plenum Press.

171 Carr, D. H. 1967. Chromosome anomalies as a cause of spontaneous abortion. *Am. J. Obstet. Gynecol.* 97(3):283.

172 Freire-Maria, N. 1970. Abortions, chromosomal aberrations and radiation. *Soc. Biol.* 17(2):102–6.

173 Hertig, A. T. 1967. The overall problem in man. In *Comparative aspects of reproductive failure*, ed. K. Benirschke, pp. 11–41. New York: Springer-Verlag.

174 Hertig, A. T., and Rock, J. 1949. A series of potentially abortive ova recovered from fertile women prior to the first missed menstrual period. *Am. J. Obstet. Gynecol.* 58:968–93.

175 Hertig, A. T.; Rock, J.; Adams, E. C.; and Menkin, M. C. 1959. Thirty-four fertilized human ova, good, bad and indifferent,

recovered from 210 women of known fertility. *Pediatrics* 23(1, part 2):202–11.

176 Jacobs, P. A. 1970. Chromosome abnormalities and population studies. In *Congenital malformations*, ed. F. C. Fraser and V. A. McKusick. Amsterdam and New York: Excerpta Medica.

177 Joel, C. A. 1967. Correlation of semen morphology with abortion and infertility. *Fertil. Steril.*, *5th World Conf.* New York: Excerpta Medica.

178 Kerr, M. G. 1971. Prenatal mortality and genetic wastage in man (a lecture). *J. Biosoc. Sci.* 3(2):223–37.

179 Lazar, P.; Gueguen, S.; Boué, J.; and Boué, A. 1973. Epidémiologie des avortements spontanés précoces: À propos de 1469 avortements caryotypés. In *Chromosomal errors in relation to reproductive failure*, ed. A. Boué and C. Thibault, pp. 317–32. Paris: I.N.S.E.R.M.

180 Lazar, P.; Guegen, S.; Boué, J.; and Boué, A. 1971. Sur la distribution des âges de 715 mères ayant eu un avortement spontané précoce. *C. R. Acad. Sci.*, ser. D, 272(22):2852–55.

181 Leridon, H., and Boué, J. 1971. La mortalité intra-utérine d'origine chromosique. *Population* 26(1):113–38.

182 Mikamo, K. 1970. Anatomic and chromosomal anomalies in spontaneous abortion. *Amer. J. Obstet. Gynecol.* 106(2):243–54.

183 Nishimura, H. 1970. Incidence of malformations in abortions. In *Congenital malformations*, pp. 275–83. International Conference Series, no. 204. Amsterdam: Excerpta Medica.

184 Pawlowitzki, I. H. 1972. Frequency of chromosome abnormalities in abortions. *Humangenetik* 16:131–36.

185 Peritz, E. 1971. A statistical study of the intrauterine selection factors related to the ABO system. II. The analysis of foetal mortality data. *Annal. Human Genet.* 34(4):382–94.

186 Poland, B. J. 1968. Study of developmental anomalies. *Am. J. Obstet. Gynecol.* 100(4):501.

187 Retel-Laurentin, A. 1967. Influence de certaines maladies sur la fécondité: Un exemple africain. *Population* 22(5):841–60.

188 Roberts, D. F., and Bonne, B. 1975. Reproduction and inbreeding among the Samaritans. *Soc. Biol.* 20(1):64–70.

189 Sentrakul, P., and Potter, E. L. 1966. Pathologic diagnosis on 2681 abortions at the Chicago Lying-in Hospital, 1957–67. *Am. J. Public Health* 56:2083–92.

190 Witschi, E. 1970. Teratogenic effects from overripeness of the egg. In *Congenital malformations*, ed. F. C. Fraser and V. A. McKusick. Amsterdam and New York: Excerpta Medica.

1.122 Perinatal Mortality

[Note: Literature on the various aspects of perinatal mortality and morbidity is abundant, and I give here only a short list of references that can be used as "entries" to other works.]

192 Butler, N. R., and Bonham, D. G. 1963. Perinatal mortality. Edinburgh: E. and S. Livingstone.
193 Butler, N. R., and Alberman, E. D. 1969. Perinatal problems. Edinburgh: E. and S. Livingstone.
194 Fischler, B., et al. 1971. On linear models in the study of perinatal mortality. *Demography* 8(3):401–10.
195 National Center for Health Statistics. 1966. *Infant, foetal, and maternal mortality.* Vital and Health Statistics, ser. 20, no. 3. Washington, D.C.: U.S. Department of Health, Education, and Welfare.
196 Janerich, D. T., et al. 1971. Season of birth and neonatal mortality. *Am. J. Public Health* 61(6):1119–25.
197 Kucera, J. 1971. Movement of the frequencies of congenital malformations in time and space. *Soc. Biol.* 18(4):422–30.
198 Potter, E. L., and Davis, M. E. 1969. Perinatal mortality. *Am. J. Obstet. Gynecol.* 105(3):335–48.
199 *Prévention de la mortalité et de la morbidité périnatales.* 1970. Série de Rapports Techniques, no. 457. Geneva: WHO.
200 Resseguie, L. J. 1973. Changes in stillbirth ratios resulting from changing fashions in age of child-bearing. *Soc. Biol.* 20(2):173–84.
201 Schlesinger, E. R., et al. 1972. Long-term trends in perinatal deaths among offspring of mothers with previous child losses. *Am. J. Epidemiol.* 96:255–62.
202 Schofield, R. S. 1970. Perinatal mortality in Hawkshead, Lancashire, 1581–1710. *Local Pop. Studies*, no. 4 (Spring) pp. 11–16.
203 Teitelbaum, M. S. 1971. Male and female components of perinatal mortality: International trends, 1901–63. *Demography* 8(4):541–48.
204 Yerushalmy, J. 1971. The relationship of parents' cigarette smoking to outcome of pregnancy: Implications as to the problem of inferring causation from observed associations. *Am. J. Epidemiol.* 93(6):443–56.

1.13 Postpartum Sterility—Breast-feeding

205 Baxi, P. J. 1957. A natural history of childbearing in the hospital class of women in Bombay. *J. Obstet. Gynecol. India* 8:26–51.
206 Bergues, H. 1948. Répercussions des calamités de guerre sur la première enfance. *Population* 3(3):501–18.
207a Bonte, M., and Van Balen, H. 1969. Prolonged lactation and family spacing in Rwanda. *J. Biosoc. Sci.* 1(2):97–100.
207b Buchanan, R. 1975. Breast-feeding: Aid to infant health and fertility control. *Pop. Rep.*, ser. J, no. 4 (July).
208 Cantrelle, P., and Leridon, H. 1971. Breast-feeding, mortality in childhood and fertility in a rural zone of Senegal. *Pop. Studies* 25(3):505–33.
209 Ginsberg, R. B. 1973. The effect of lactation on the length of the post-partum anovulatory period: An application of a bivariate stochastic model. *Theor. Pop. Biol.* 4(3):276–99.
210 Henry, L. 1964. Mesure du temps mort en fécondité naturelle. *Population* 19(3):485–514.

211 Jain, A. K. 1969. Pregnancy outcome and the time required for next conception. *Pop. Studies* 23(3):421–33.
212 Jain, A. K.; Hsu, T. C.; Freedman, R.; and Chang, M. C. 1970. Demographic aspects of lactation and post-partum amenorrhea. *Demography* 7(2):255–71.
213 Jain, A. K., and Sun, T. H. 1972. Inter-relationship between socio-demographic factors, lactation and post-partum amenorrhea. *Demography India* 1(1):1–15.
214 Jelliffe, D. B., and Jelliffe, E. F. P. 1972. Lactation, conception and the nutrition of the nursing mother and child. *J. Pediat.* 81:829–33.
215 Knodel, J. 1968. Infant mortality and fertility in three Bavarian villages: An analysis of family histories from the 19th century. *Pop. Studies* 22(3):297–318.
216 Knodel, J., and Van de Walle, E. 1967. Breast-feeding, fertility and infant mortality: An analysis of some early German data. *Pop. Studies* 21(2):109–31.
217 Koh, K. S., and Smith, D. P. 1970. *The National Survey on Fertility and Family Planning, 1968.* Rep. of Korea: National Family Planning Center, Ministry of Health.
218 Leroy-Ladurie, E. 1969. L'aménorrhée de famine (XVIIème-XXème siècle). *Annales E.S.C.* 24(6):1589–1601.
219 Pascal, J. 1969. Quelque aspects de la physiologie du post-partum. Thèse pour le Doctorat en Médecine, Nancy. (See note by H. Leridon in *Population* 30[1]:117–20.)
220 Perez, A.; Vela, P.; Masnick, G.; and Potter, R. G. 1972. First ovulation after childbirth: The effect of breast-feeding. *Am. J. Obstet. Gynecol.* 114(8):1041–47.
221 Perez, A.; Vela, P.; Potter, R. G.; and Masnick, G. 1971. Timing and sequence of resuming ovulation and menstruation after childbirth. *Pop. Studies* 25(3):491–503.
222 Philippe, P. 1974. Amenorrhea, intrauterine mortality and parental consanguinity in an isolated French Canadian population. *Human Biol.* 46(3):405–24.
224 Potter, R. G.; Wyon, J.; New, M.; and Gordon, J. 1965. Applications of field studies to research on the physiology of human reproduction (lactation and its effects upon birth intervals in eleven Punjab villages). *J. Chronic Diseases* 18:1125–40.
225 Salber, E.; Feinleib, M., and MacMahon, B. 1966. The duration of post-partum amenorrhea. *Am. J. Epidemiol.* 82(3):347–58.
226 Sharman, A. 1951. Ovulation after pregnancy. *Fertil. Steril.* 2:371–93.
227 Sharman, A. 1967. Ovulation in the post-partum period. *Int. J. Fertil.* 12(1):14–16.
228 Stein, Z. and Susser, M. 1975. Fertility, fecundity, famine: Food rations in the Dutch famine 1944/5 have a causal relation to fertility, and probably to fecundity. *Human Biol.* 47(1):131–54.

229 Tietze, C. 1961. The effect of breast-feeding on the rate of conception. *International Population Conference*, New York. 2:129–36. London: I.U.S.S.P.
230 van de Walle, E., and van de Walle, F. 1972. Allaitement, stérilité et contraception: Les opinions jusqu'au XIXème siècle. *Population* 27(4–5):685–702.
231 Van Ginneken, J. K. 1974. Prolonged breastfeeding as a birth spacing method. *Stud. Fam. Plan.*, 5(6):201–6.

1.14 Permanent and Temporary Sterility

232 Joel, C. A., ed. 1971. *Fertility disturbances in men and women*. Basel: S. Kärger.
233 Freedman, R.; Whelpton, P. K.; and Campbell, A. 1959. Family planning, sterility, and population growth. New York: McGraw-Hill.
234 Harter, C. L. 1970: The fertility of sterile and subfecund women in New Orleans. *Soc. Biol.* 17(3):195–206.
235 Henry, L. 1953. *Fécondité des marriages: Nouvelle méthode de mesure*. Travaux et Documents, no. 16. Paris: I.N.E.D.–P.U.F. Chaps. 6, 7.
236 Hervet, E., and Barrat, J. 1968. Stérilité—Contraception. Paris: Baillière et Fils.
237 Leridon, H. 1971. Fécondité, stérilité et types d'unions. *Cah. O.R.S.T.O.M.*, *Ser. Sci. Hum.* 8(1):91–96.
238 McFalls, J. A. 1973. Impact of VD on the fertility of the U.S. black population. *Soc. Biol.* 20(1):2–19.
239 Pittenger, D. B. 1973. An exponential model of female sterility. *Demography* 10(1):113–21.
240 Retel-Laurentin, A. 1967. Influence de certaines maladies sur la fécondité: Un exemple africain. *Population* 22(5):841–60.
241 Romaniuk, A. 1968. L'infécondité en Afrique tropicale. In *La population de l'Afrique tropicale*. New York: Population Council.
242 Stoeckel, J.; Chowdhury, A. K.; and Mosley, W. H. 1972. The effect of fecundity on fertility in rural East Pakistan. *Soc. Biol.* 19(2):193–201.
243 Vincent, P. 1950. La stérilité physiologique des populations. *Population* 5(1):45–64.
244 Weir, W. C., and Weir, D. R. 1961. The natural history of infertility. *Fertil. Steril.* 12:443–51.

1.2 Characteristics of Births

1.21 Sex

245 Bernstein, M. E. 1958. A genetic explanation of the wartime increase in the secondary sex-ratio. *Am. J. Human Genet.* 10(1):68–70.
246 Bernstein, M. E. 1970. Interrelations between paternal age and the human sex ratio: A confirmation of E. Novitski's theorem. *Genus* 26(1–2):251–58.
247 Bodmer, W. F., and Edward, A. W. 1960. Natural selection and the sex-ratio. *Ann. Human Genet.* 24:239–44.

248 Goodman, L. A. 1961. Some possible effects of birth control on the human sex-ratio. *Ann. Human Genet.* 25:75–81.

249 Haldar, A. K., and Bhattacharya, N. 1970. Fertility and sex-sequence of children of Indian couples. *Rech. écon. Louvain* vol. 36, no. 4 (Nov.).

250 Novitski, E., and Kimball, A. W., 1958. Birth order, parental ages, and sex of offspring. *Am. J. Human Genet.* 10(3):268–75.

251 Novitski, E., and Sandlers, L. 1956. The relationship between parental age, birth order and the secondary sex-ratio in humans. *Ann. Human Genet.* 21:123–31.

252 Pakrasi, K., and Halder, A. 1971. Sex ratios and sex sequences of births in India. *J. Biosoc. Sci.* 3(4):377–88.

253 Robinson, H., and Masi, A. T. 1972. The use of the binominal distribution to ascertain bias in studies involving the sex ratio. *Human Biol.* 44(1):1–13.

254 Slatis, H. M. 1953. Seasonal variations in the American live birth sex ratio. *Am. J. Human Genet.* 5(1):21–33.

255 Teitelbaum, M. S. 1970. Factors affecting the sex-ratio in large populations. *J. Biosoc. Sci.* 2(supp. 2):61–71.

256 Teitelbaum, M. S. 1971. Male and female components of perinatal mortality: International trends, 1901–63. *Demography* 8(4):541–48.

257 Teitelbaum, M. S., and Mantel, N. 1971. Socio-economic factors and the sex-ratio at birth. *J. Biosoc. Sci.* 3(1):23–42.

258 Tricomi, V.; Serr, D.; and Solish, G. 1960. The ratio of male to female embryos as determined by the sex-chromatine. *Am. J. Obstet. Gynecol.* 79(3):504.

1.22 Multiple Births

259 Darnaud, F. 1975. Données récentes sur les accouchements multiples. *Population* 30(3):551–68.

260 Gittelsohn, A., and Milham, S. 1964. Statistical study of twins: Methods. *Am. J. Pub. Health* 54(2):286–94.

261 Guttmacher, A. F. 1953. The incidence of multiple births in man and some of the other unipara. *Obstet. Gynceol.* 2(1):22–35.

262 Heuser, R. L. 1967. Multiple Births: United States, 1964. N.C.H.S. Vital and Health Statistics, series 21, no. 14. Washington, D.C.: U.S. Department of Health, Education and Welfare.

263 James, W. H. 1972. Secular changes in dizygotic twinning rates. *J. Biosoc. Sci.* 4(4):427–34.

264 Zeleny, C. 1921. The relative number of twins and triplets. *Science* 53:262–63.

1.23 Anomalies

265 Carter, C. O. 1973. Nature and distribution of genetic abnormalities. *J. Biosoc. Sci.* 5(2):261–72.

266 *Congenital malformations: Proceedings of the third international conference, The Hague, the Netherlands, 1969*, ed. F. C. Fraser and V. A. McKusick. Amsterdam: Excerpta Medica.

267 Cruz-Coke, R.; Valenzuela, Y.; and Navaro, J. 1972. La morbidité génétique: Méthodes de mesures et résultats obtenus à Santiago. *Population* 27(6):1045–52.

268 Smith, C. A. B. 1972. Note on the estimation of parental age effects. *Ann. Human Genet.* 35(3):337–42.

269 Wilson, J. G. 1973. Environment and birth defects. New York: Academic Press.

270 World Health Organization. Special Subject: Congenital malformations (1961–67). 1971. *World Health Stat. Rep.* 24(11):657–713.

1.4 Models

271 Barrett, J. C. 1969. A Monte-Carlo simulation of human reproduction. *Genus* 25:1–22.

272 Barrett, J. C. 1971. Use of a fertility simulation model to refine measurement techniques. *Demography* 8(4):481–90.

273 Basu, D. 1955. A note on the structure of a stochastic model considered by V. M. Dandekar. *Sankhya* 15:251–52.

274 Bodmer, W. F., and Jacquard, A. 1968. La variance de la dimension des familles selon divers facteurs de la fécondité. *Population* 23(5):869–78.

275 Bogaarts, J. 1976. Intermediate fertility variables and marital fertility rates *Pop. Studies* 30(2):227–42.

276 Brass, W. 1958. The distribution of births in human populations. *Pop. Studies* 12:51–72.

277a Chiang, C. L. 1968. Introduction to stochastic processes in biostatistics. New York: John Wiley and Sons.

277b Coale, A. J., and Trussell, T. J. 1974. Model fertility schedules: Variations in the age structure of childbearing in human populations. *Pop. Index* 40(2):185–258.

278 Dyke, B., and MacCluer, J. W., eds. 1973. *Computer simulation in human population studies*. New York: Academic Press.

279a Dandekar, V. M. 1955. Certain modified forms of binomial and Poisson distributions. *Sankhya* 15:237–50.

279b Das Gupta, P. 1973. A stochastic model of human reproduction: Some preliminary results. *J. Theor. Pop. Biol.* 4:466–90.

280 Dharmadhikari, S. W. 1964. A generalization of a stochastic model considered by V. M. Dandekar. *Sankhya* Ser. A, 26:31–38.

281 Heer, D., and Smith, D. 1968. Mortality level, desired family size, and population increase. *Demography* 5(1):104–21.

282 Henry, L. 1957. Fécondité et famille: Modèles mathématiques. *Population* 12(3):413–44.

283 Henry, L. 1961. Fécondité et famille: Modèles mathématiques. II. *Population* 16(1):27–48.

284 Henry, 1961. Fécondité et famille: Modèles mathématiques. III: applications numériques. *Population* 16(2):261–82.
285 Henry, L. 1953. Fondements théoriques des mesures de la fécondité naturelle. *Revue Inst. Intern. Stat.* 21(3):135–51.
286 Henry, L. 1972. On the measurement of human fertility, ed. M. C. Sheps and E. Lapierre-Adamcyk. New York: Elsevier.
287 Hoem, J. M. 1968. *A probabilistic model for primary marital fertility.* Oslo: Statistik Sentralbyra.
288 Hoem, J. M. 1968. Fertility rates and reproduction rates in a probabilistic setting. Oslo: Statistik Sentralbyra.
289 Holmberg, I. 1968. Demography models. Reports 8. Göteborg: Demographic Institute.
290 Holmberg, I. 1970, 1972. Fecundity, fertility and family planning: Application of demographic micromodels. Reports 10, 11. Göteborg: Demographic Institute.
291 Horvitz, D. G.; Giebsrecht, F. G.; Shah, B. V.; and Lachenbruch, P. A. 1971. POPSIM, a demographic microsimulation model. Congrès de Londres (1969), 1:95–106. Liège: U.I.E.S.P.
292 Hyrenius, H., and Adolfsson, I. 1964. A fertility simulation model. (DM 1). Reports 2. Göteborg: Demographic Institute.
293 Hyrenius, H.; Adolfsson, I.; Holmberg, I. 1966. Demographic models, Second Report (DM 2). Reports 4. Göteborg: Demographic Institute.
294 Hyrenius, H.; Holmberg, I.; and Carlsson, M. 1967. Demographic models. (DM 3). Reports 5. Göteborg: Demographic Institute.
295 Jacquard, A. 1967. La reproduction humaine en régime malthusien: Un modèle de simulation par la méthode de Monte-Carlo. *Population* 22(5):897–920.
296 Jacquard, A., and Leridon, H. 1973. Simulating human reproduction: How complicated should a model be? In *Computer simulation in human population studies*, ed. B. Dyke and J. MacCluer. New York: Academic Press.
297 Khalifa, A. M. 1972. Towards a computerized demographic micro-simulation model for Egypt: Experimentation of POPSIM (I). *Egypt. Pop. Fam. Plan. Rev.* 5(2):153–66.
298 Khalifa, A. M., and Rachad, H. 1972. A model for human reproduction: The case of Egypt. *Egypt. Pop. Fam. Plan. Rev.* 5(2):99–114.
300 Leridon, H., and Henry, L. 1968. Influence du calendrier de la contraception. *Population* 23(6):1009–54.
301 Lombardo, E. 1968. Un modello di riproduzione di una coorte umana in Italia: Simulazione stocastica. *Genus* 24:177–207.
302 Mode, C. 1974. Applications of computerized stochastic models of human reproduction and population growth in family planning evaluation. *Math. Biosci.* 20:267–92.
303 Perrin, E. B., and Sheps, M. C. 1964. Human reproduction: a stochastic process. *Biometrics* 20:28–45.

304 Pollard, J. H. 1969. A discrete-time two-sex age specific stochastic population program incorporating marriage. *Demography* 6(2): 185–221.

305 Potter, R. G.; Jain, A. K.; and McCann, B. 1970. Net delay of next conception by contraception: A highly simplified case. *Pop. Studies* 24(2):173–92.

306 Potter, R. G., and Sakoda, J. 1966. A computer model of family building based on expected values. *Demography* 3(2):450–61.

307 Potter, R. G., and Sakoda, J. 1967. Family Planning and fecundity. *Pop. Studies* 20(3):311–28.

308 Potter, R. G.; Sakoda, J.; and Feinberg, W. 1968 Variable fecundability and the timing of births. *Eugenics Quart.* 15(3):155–63.

309 Ridley, J. C., and Sheps, M. C. 1966. An analytic simulation model of human reproduction with demographic and biological components. *Pop. Studies* 19(3):297–310.

310 Ridley, J. C.; Sheps, M. C.; Lingner, J. W.; and Menken, J. A. 1969. On the apparent subfecundity of non-family planners. *Soc. Biol.* 16:24–28.

311 Sheps, M. C. 1965. Applications of probability models to the study of patterns of human reproduction. In *Public health and population change*, ed. M. C. Sheps and J. C. Ridley. Pittsburgh: University of Pittsburg Press.

312 Sheps, M. C. 1971. A review of models for population change. *Rev. Int. Inst. Stat.* 39(2):185–96.

313 Sheps, M. C., and Menken, J. A. 1973. *Mathematical models of conception and birth*. Chicago: University of Chicago Press.

314 Sheps, M. C.; Menken, J. A.; and Radick, A. P. 1969. Probability models for family building: an analytical review. *Demography* 6(2): 161–83.

315 Sheps, M. C., and Perrin, E. B. 1963. Changes in birth rates as a function of contraceptive effectiveness: Some applications of a stochastic model. *Am. J. Public Health* 53:1031–46.

316 Siegel, J., and Akers, D. 1969. Some aspects of the use of birth expectations data from sample surveys for population projections. *Demography* 6(2):101–15.

317 Singh, S. N. 1964. A probability model for couple fertility. *Sankhya, Ser. B*, 26:89–94.

318 Singh, S. N., and Bhattacharya, B. N. 1970. A generalized probability distribution for couple fertility. *Biometrics* 26:33–40.

319 Venkatacharya, K. 1969. An examination of a certain bias to truncation in the context of simulation models of human reproduction. *Sankhya,* ser. B, 31(3–4):397–412.

320 Venkatacharya, K. 1972. Reduction in fertility due to induced abortions: A simulation model. *Demography* 9(3):339–52.

321 Venkatacharya, K. 1970. Some implications of susceptibility and its application in fertility evaluation models. *Sankhya,* ser. B, 32:41–54.

1.5 Data on Natural Fertility

322 Cantrelle, P. 1969. *Etude démographique dans la région du Siné-Saloum (Sénégal)* Paris: O.R.S.T.O.M.

323 Charbonneau, H. 1970. *Tourouvre-au-Perche aux XVIIème et XVIIIème siècles: Etude de démographie historique.* Travaux et Documents, no. 55. Paris: I.N.E.D.–P.U.F.

324 Cross, H. E., and McKusick, V. A. 1970. Amish demography. *Soc. Biol.* 17(2):83–101.

325 Dandekar, K. 1959. Demographic survey of six rural communities. Bombay: Gokhale Institute of Politics and Economics. (See comment by L. Henry in *Population* 15(1):144–147 (Jan. 1960).)

326 Deniel, R., and Henry, L. 1965. La population d'un village du nord de la France, Sainghin-en-Mélantois, de 1665 à 1851. *Population* 20(4): 563–602.

327 Eaton, J. W., and Mayer, A. J. 1954. *Man's capacity to reproduce: The demography of a unique population.* Glencoe, Ill.: Free Press.

328a Eaton, J. W., and Mayer, A. J. 1953. The social biology of very high fertility among the Hutterites: The demography of a unique population. *Human Biol.* 25(3):206–64.

328b Ferry, B. 1977. *Etude de la fécondité à Dakar (Sénégal).* Travaux et Documents. Paris: O.R.S.T.O.M.

329 Frezel-Lozey, M. 1969. Histoire démographique d'un village en Béarn: Bilhères-d'Ossau (XVIIIème–XIXème siècle). Bordeaux: Biscaye Frères, Imp.

330 Ganiage, J. 1960. La population européenne de Tunis au milieu du XIXème siècle. Paris: P.U.F.

331 Ganiage, J. 1963. Trois villages de l'Ile-de-France au XVIIème siècle: Etude démographique. Travaux et Documents, no. 40. Paris: I.N.E.D.–P.U.F.

332 Gautier, E., and Henry, L. 1958. La population de Crulai, paroisse normande: étude historique. Travaux et Documents, no. 33. Paris: I.N.E.D.–P.U.F.

333 Girard, P. 1959. Aperçus de la démographie de Sotteville-lès-Rouen vers la fin du XVIIIème siècle. *Population* 14(3):485–508.

334 Henripin, J. 1954. La fécondité des ménages canadiens au début du XVIIIème siècle. *Population* 9(1):61–84.

335 Henripin, J. 1954. La population canadienne au début du XVIIIème siècle. Travaux et Documents, no. 22. Paris: I.N.E.D.–P.U.F.

336 Henry, L. 1956. Anciennes familles genevoises: Etude démographique, XVIéme–XXème siècles. Travaux et Documents, no. 26. Paris: I.N.E.D.–P.U.F.

337 Henry, L. 1972. Fécondité des mariages dans le quart sud-ouest de la France de 1720 à 1829. *Annales E.S.C.* 27(3):612–39; 27(4–5): 977–1023.

338 Henry, L. 1961. La fécondité naturelle: Observations, théorie, résultat. *Population* 16(4):625–36.

339 Henry, L. 1970. La population de la Norvège depuis deux siècles. *Population* 25(3):543–58.

340 Henry, L. 1961. Some data on natural fertility. *Eugenics Quart.* 8(2): 81–91.

341 Henry, L., and Houdaille, J. 1973. La fécondité dans le quart nord-ouest de la France, de 1670 à 1829. *Population* 28(4–5):873–924.

342 Hollingsworth, T. H. 1964. The demography of the British peerage. *Population Studies*, suppl. vol. 18, no. 2.

343 Houdaille, J. 1967. La population de Boulay (Moselle) avant 1850. *Population* 22(6):1055–84.

344 Houdaille J., 1971. La population de sept villages des environs de Boulay (Moselle) aux XVIIIème et XIXème siècles. *Population* 26(6): 1061–72.

345 Hyrenius, H. 1958. Fertility and reproduction in a Swedish population group without family limitation. *Pop. Studies* 12(2):121–30.

346 Knodel, J. 1970. Two and a half centuries of demographic history in a Bavarian village. *Pop. Studies* 24(3):353–76.

347 Lachiver, M. 1969. La population de Meulan du XVIIème au XIXème siècle (1600–1870). Paris: S.E.V.P.E.N.

348 Leridon, H. 1971. Les facteurs de la fécondité en Martinique. *Population* 26(2):277–300.

349 Leridon, H.; Zucker, E.; and Cazenave, M. 1970. *Fécondité et famille en Martinique: Faits, attitudes, opinions.* Travaux et Documents, no. 56. Paris: I.N.E.D.–P.U.F.

350 Lorimer, F., et al. 1954. *Culture and human fertility.* Paris: U.N.E.S.C.O.

351 Okasaki, A. 1951. *Fertility of the farming population in Japan.* Tokyo: Research Institute of Population Problems.

352 Potter, R. G.; New, M. L.; Wyon, J. B.; and Gordon, J. E. 1965. A fertility differential in Eleven Punjab villages. *Milbank Mem. Fund Quart.* 43(2):185–201.

353 Sheps, M. C. 1965. An analysis of reproductive patterns in an American Isolate. *Pop. Studies* 19(1):65–80.

354 Smith, D. S. 1974. A homeostatic demographic regime: Patterns in West European family reconstitution studies. Philadelphia: Conference on Behavioral Models in Historical Demography.

355 Smith, T. E. 1960. The Cocos-Keeling Islands: A demographic laboratory. *Pop. Studies* 14(2):91–130.

356 *Statistique générale du mouvement de la population, 1749–1905.* 1907. Paris: Statistique générale de la France.

357 Tietze, C. 1957. Reproductive span and rate of reproduction among Hutterite women. *Fertil. Steril.* 8(1):89–97.

358 Valmary, P. 1965. Familles paysannes au XVIIIème siècle en Bas-Quercy: Etude démographique. Travaux et Documents, no. 45. Paris: I.N.E.D.–P.U.F.

359 Vincent, P. 1961. Recherches sur la fécondité biologique: Etude d'un groupe de familles nombreuses. Travaux et Documents, no. 37. Paris: I.N.E.D.–P.U.F.

360 Wrigley, E. A. 1966. Family limitation in pre-industrial England. *Econ. Hist. Rev.*, 2d ser. 19(1):82–109.

361 Wyon, J. B., and Gordon, J. E. 1971. The Khanna study: Population problems in the rural Punjab. Cambridge: Harvard University Press.

2 The Control of Fertility

2.2 Methods (Contraception, Abortion, Sterilization)

2.20 General Studies

362 *Advanced concepts in contraception.* 1968. Proceedings of four symposia ed. F. Hoffman. Amsterdam: Excerpta Medica.

363 Borell, U. 1971. Side-effects of fertility controlling agents. In *Control of human fertility*, ed. E. Diczfalusy and U. Borell. Proceedings of the 15th Nobel Symposium, Lidingo, Sweden, 1970. New York: Wiley.

364a Diczfalusy, E., and Borell, U., eds. 1971. *Control of human fertility.* Proceedings of the 15th Nobel Symposium, Lidingo, Sweden, 1970. New York: Wiley.

364b Freedman, R., and Takeshita, J. Y. 1969. *Family Planning in Taiwan: An experiment in social change.* Princeton: Princeton University Press.

365 Himes, N. E. 1963. *Medical history of contraception.* 2d ed. New York: Gamut Press.

366 Loraine, J. E., and Bell, E. T. 1968. Fertility and contraception in the human female. Edinburgh and London: E. and S. Livingstone.

367 Pearl, R. 1932. Contraception and fertility in 2,000 women. *Human Biol.* 4:363–407.

367b Ross, J. A.; Germain, A.; Forrest, J. E.; and Van Ginneken, J. 1972. Findings from family planning research. *Reports on population/Family Planning*, 12 Oct.

368 Ryder, N. B. 1973. Contraceptive failure in the United States. *Fam. Plan. Perspect.* 5(3):133–42.

369 Sivin, I. 1974. *Contraception and fertility change in the international postpartum program.* New York: Population Council.

370 Tietze, C. 1965. *Effectiveness, acceptability, and safety of modern contraceptive methods.* New York: National Committee on Maternal Health.

371 *Methods of fertility regulation: Advances in research and clinical experience.* Technical Report Series, no. 473. Geneva: WHO.

2.22 Rhythm (Calendar and Temperature)

372*a* Barrett, J., and Marshall, J. 1969. The risk of conception on different days of the menstrual cycle. *Pop. Studies* 23(3):455–61.

372*b* *Biology of fertility control by periodic abstinence.* 1967. Technical Report Series, no. 360. Geneva: WHO.

373 Brayer, F. T.; Chiazze, L.; and Duffy, B. J. 1969. Calendar rhythm and menstrual cycle range. *Fertil. Steril.* 20(9):279–88.

374 James, W. H. 1965. Parameters of the menstrual cycle and the efficiency of rhythm method of contraception. *Pop. Studies* 19(1):45–64.

375 Potter, R. G. 1966. Parameters of the menstrual cycle: A reply. *Pop. Studies* 20(2):223–32.

376 Potter, R. G.; Burch, T. K.; and Matsumoto, S. 1967. Long cycles, late ovulation, and calendar rhythm. *Int. J. Fertil.* 12(1, part 2): 127–40.

377 Potter, R. G.; Sagi, P. C.; and Westoff, C. F. 1962. Knowledge of the ovulatory cycle and coital frequency as factors affecting conception and contraception. *Milbank Mem. Fund Quart.* 40(1):46–58.

378 Ross, C., and Piotrow, P. T. 1974. Birth control without contraceptives. *Pop. Rep.*, ser. A, no. 1. George Washington University.

379 Tietze, C.; Poliakoff, S.; and Rock, J. 1951. The clinical effectiveness of the rhythm method of contraception. *Fertil. Steril.* 2(5):444–50.

380 Tietze, C., and Potter, R. G. 1962. Statistical evaluation of the rhythm method. *Am. J. Obstet. Gynecol.* 84(5):692–98.

381 Vincent, B. 1967. *Méthode thermique et contraception: Approches médicale et psycho-sociologique.* Paris: Masson.

2.24 Oral Contraceptives

382 *Hormonal steroids in contraception.* 1968. Technical Report Series, no. 386. Geneva: WHO.

385 James, W. H. 1971. Coital rates and the pill. *Nature* 234:555–56.

386 Piotrow, P. T., and Lee, C. M. 1974. Oral contraceptives: 50 million users. *Pop. Rep.*, Ser. A, no. 1.

387 Potts, M., et al. 1975. Advantages of orals outweigh disadvantages. *Pop. Rep.*, ser. A, no. 2.

388 Ravenholt, R. T.; Piotrow, P. T.; and Speidel, J. J. 1970. Use of oral contraceptives: A decade of controversy. *Int. J. Gynaecol. Obstet.* 8(6, ii):941–56.

389 Westoff, C., and Ryder, N. B. 1968. Duration of use of oral contraception in the United States, 1960–65. *Pub. Health Rep.* 83(4):277–87.

2.25 Intrauterine Devices

390 Bernard, R. P. 1970. I.U.D. performance patterns: A 1970 world view. *Int. J. Gynaec. Obstet.* 8(6, ii):926–40.

391 Huber, S. C., et al. 1975. I.U.D. reassessed: A decade of experience. *Pop. Rep.*, ser. B, no. 2. George Washington University.

392 *Intrauterine devices: Physiological and clinical aspects.* 1968. Technical Report Series, no. 397. Geneva: WHO

393 Lewit, S. 1970. Outcome of pregnancy with intrauterine devices. *Contraception* 2(1):47–57.

394 Snowden, R.; Eckstein, P.; and Hawkins, D. 1973. Social and medical factors in the use and effectiveness of IUDs. *J. Biosoc. Sci.* 5(1): 31–49.

395 *Report on intrauterine contraceptive devices.* 1968. Washington, D.C.: Advisory Committee on Obstetrics and Gynecology, Food and Drug Administration.

396 Tietze, C., and Lewit, S. 1971. The IUD and the pill: Extended use-effectiveness. *Family Plan. Perspect.* 3(2):53–55.

397 Wheeler, R. G.; Duncan, G. W.; and Speidel, J. J., eds. 1974. *Intrauterine devices: Development, evaluation, and program implementation.* New York: Academic Press.

2.28 Abortion

398 *Abortion, obtained and denied: Research approaches.* 1971. New York: Population Council.

399 Coombs, L.; Freedman, R.; and Namboothiri, D. N. 1969. Inferences about abortion from foetal mortality data. *Pop. Studies* 23(2): 247–65.

400 Floyd, M. K. 1973. *Abortion bibliography*, 1972. Troy, N.Y.: Whitston Publ. Co.

401 Hordern, A. 1971. *Legal abortion: The English experience* (with a foreword by Brudenell). Oxford: Pergamon Press.

402a Klinger, A. 1970. Demographic consequences of the legalization of induced abortion in Eastern Europe. *Int. J. Gynaecol. Obstet.* 8(52): 680–91.

402b Potter, R. G.; Ford, K.; and Moots, B. 1975. Competition between spontaneous and induced abortion. *Demography* 12(1):129–41.

403a Tietze, C. 1970. Induced abortion as a method of fertility control. In *Fertility and family planning: A world review*, ed. S. J. Behrman, L. Corsa, and R. Freedman. Ann Arbor: University of Michigan Press.

403b Williams, S. J., and Pullum, T. W. 1975. Effectiveness of abortion as birth control. *Soc. Biol.* 22:23–33.

2.29 Sterilization

404 Bumpass, L. L., and Presser, H. B. 1972. Contraceptive sterilization in the U.S.: 1965 and 1970. *Demography* 9(4):531–48.

405 Haynes, M. A., et al. 1969. A study on the effectiveness of sterilization in reducing the birth rate. *Demography* 6(1):1–12.

406 Presser, H. B. 1970. Voluntary sterilization: A world view. *Reports on Population, Family Planning*, no. 5 (July).

407 Presser, H. B. 1969. The role of sterilization in controlling Puerto-Rican fertility. *Pop. Studies* 23(3):343–61.

408 Pratt, W. 1975. The practice of sterilization in the United States: Preliminary findings of the 1973 National Survey of Family Growth. Annual meeting of the P.A.A., Seattle, April 1975.

409 Presser, H. B., and Bumpass, L. L. 1972. The acceptability of contraceptive sterilization among US couples, 1970. *Fam. Plan. Perspect.* 4(4):18–28.

410 Wortman, J., and Piotrow, P. T. 1973. Vasectomy: Old and new techniques. *Pop. Rep.* ser. D, no. 1. George Washington University.

2.3 Measurement of Effectiveness

2.31 Effectiveness: Individual Level

411 Gini, C. 1942. Sur la mesure de l'efficacité des pratiques anticonceptionnelles. *Rev. I.I.S.* 10(1–2):1–36.

412 Henry, L. 1968. Essai de calcul de l'efficacité de la contraception. *Population* 23(2):265–78.

413 Jain, A. K. 1969. Relative fecundability of users and non-users of contraception. *Soc. Biol.* 16(1):39–43.

414 Pearl, R. 1932. Contraception and fertility in 2000 women. *Human Biology* 4(3):363–407.

415 Potter, R. G. 1966. Application of life table techniques to measurement of contraceptive effectiveness. *Demography* 3(2):297–304.

416 Potter, R. G. 1960. Length of the observation period as a factor affecting the contraceptive failure rate. *Milbank Mem. Fund Quart.* 38(2):140–52.

417 Potter, R. G. 1959. Some problems in predicting a couple's contraceptive future. *Eugenics Quart.* 6(4):254–59.

418 Potter, R. G. 1967. The multiple decrement life table as an approach to the measurement of use-effectiveness and demographic effectiveness of contraception. *Sydney Conference, I.U.S.S.P.*, pp. 869–83.

419 Potter, R. G.; McCann, B.; and Sakoda, J. M. 1970. Selective fecundability and contraceptive effectiveness. *Milbank Mem. Fund Quart.* 48(1):91–102.

420 Potter, R. G.; Jain, A. K.; and McCann, B. 1970. Net delay of next conception by contraception: A highly simplified case. *Pop. Studies* 24(2):173–92.

421 Potter, R. G.; Sagi, P. C.; and Westoff, C. F. 1962. Improvement of contraception during the course of marriage. *Pop. Studies* 16(2):160–74.

422 Seklani, M. 1963. Efficacité de la contraception: Méthodes et résultats. *Population* 18(2):329–48.

423 Stix, R. K., and Notestein, F. W. 1940. Controlled fertility: An evaluation of clinic service. Baltimore: Williams and Wilkins.

424 Tietze, 1959. Differential fecundity and effectiveness of contraception. *Eugenics Rev.* 50(4):231–37.

425 Tietze, C. 1962. The use-effectiveness of contraceptive methods. In *Research in family planning*, ed. C. V. Kiser, pp. 357–69. Princeton: Princeton University Press.

426 Tietze, C. 1971. Effectiveness of contraceptive methods. In *Control of human fertility*, ed. E. Diczfalusy and U. Borell. Proceedings of the 15th Nobel Symposium, Lidingo, Sweden, 1970. New York: Wiley.

427 Tietze, C., and Lewit, S. 1973. Recommended procedures for the statistical evaluation of intrauterine contraception. *Studies Fam. Plan.* 4(2):35–41.

428 Tietze, C., and Lewit, S. 1968. Statistical evaluation of contraceptive methods: Use-effectiveness and extended use-effectiveness. *Demography* 5(2):931–40.

2.32 Demographic Effectiveness

429 Barrett, J. C. 1972. The time response in averted births. *Pop. Studies* 26(3):507–14.

430 Bean, L. L., and Seltzer, W. 1968. Couple-years of protection and birth prevented: A methodological examination. *Demography* 5(2): 947–59.

431 Chang, M. C.; Liu, T. H.; and Chow, L. P. 1969. Study by matching of the demographic impact of an I.U.D. programme (Taiwan). *Milbank Mem. Fund Quart.* 47(2):137–57.

432 Chow, L. P.; Chang, M. C.; and Liu, T. H. 1969. Demographic impact of an I.U.D. programme. *Studies Fam. Plan.* 1(45):1–6.

433 Chandrasekaran, C., ed. *The demographic impact of family planning programmes.* 1975. Liège: I.U.S.S.P. and Ordina Editions.

434 Enke, D., and O'Hara, D. J. 1969. Estimating fertility changes from birth control measures. *Studies Fam. Plan.* 1(46):1–5.

435 Keyfitz, N. 1971. How birth control affects births. *Soc. Biol.* 18(2): 109–21.

436 Lee, B. M., and Isbister, J. 1966. The impact of birth control programs on fertility. In *Family planning and population programs*, ed. B. Berelson et al. Chicago: University of Chicago Press.

437a Mauldin, P. 1967. Measurement and evaluation of National Family Programs. *Demography* 4(1):71–80.

437b Nortman, D., and Bongaarts, J. 1975. Contraceptive practice required to meet a prescribed crude birth rate target: A proposed macro-model (TABRAP) and hypothetical illustrations. *Demography* 12(3): 471–92.

438 Potter, R. G. 1970. Births averted by contraception: An approach through renewal theory. *Theoret. Pop. Biol.* 1(3):251–72.

439   Potter, R. G. 1972. Contraceptive impact over several generations. In *Population Dynamics*, ed. T. N. Greville. New York: Academic Press.

440   Potter, R. G. 1969. Estimating births averted in a family planning program. In *Fertility and family planning: A world view*, ed. S. J. Behrman et al. Ann Arbor: University of Michigan Press.

442   Potter, R. G. 1971. Inadequacy of a one-method family planning program. *Studies Fam. Plan.* 2(1):1–6.

443   Potter, R. G. 1970. *A technical appendix on procedures used in manuscript: Estimating births averted in a family planning program.* Ann Arbor: Population Studies Center, University of Michigan.

444   Potter, R. G.; Masnick, G. S.; and Gendell, M. 1973. Postamenorrheic versus post-partum strategies of contraception. *Demography* 10(1):99–112.

445   Reynolds, J. 1972. Evaluation of family planning program performance: A critical review. *Demography* 9(1):69–86.

446   Sheps, M. C. 1966. Contributions of natality models to program planning and evaluation. *Demography* 3(2):445–49.

447a   Sheps, M. C., and Perrin, E. B. 1963. Changes in birth rates as a function of contraceptive effectiveness: Some applications of a stochastic model. *Am. J. Public Health* 53(7):1031–46.

447b   *Some techniques for measuring the impact of contraception.* 1974. Asian Population Studies Series, no. 18. New York: United Nations (ESCAP).

448   Tietze, C., and Bongaarts, J. 1975. Fertility rates and abortion rates: Simulations of family limitation. *Stud. Fam. Plan.* 6(5):114–20.

449   Venkatacharya, K. 1971. A model to estimate births averted due to IUCDs and sterilization. *Demography* 8(4):491–505.

450   Wolfers, D. 1969. The demographic effects of a contraceptive programme. *Pop. Studies* 23(1):111–40.

2.4   Models

(See 1.4.)

Index

Abortion: induced, as biasing data on spontaneous abortion, 48–49, 76; induced, as a birth control method, 121, 127–28, 134; induced, bibliography of, 194; late vs. early, 76; spontaneous (*see* Intrauterine mortality)

Acceptability of contraception, 122, 127

Acceptors of a family planning program, 129–30

A-conception, 151, 153

Adolescent sterility, 8–9

Amenorrhea: after hormonal contraception, 40; effect of nutrition on, 93; postpartum (*see* Nonsusceptible period following conception)

Anomalies, chromosomal, 1, 45, 76–78; bibliography of, 181–82

Anovulatory cycles: after hormonal contraception, 40; during fecund life, 14, 93–94, 103; postpartum, 40, 83–84

Apparent fecundability, 22, 35

Artificial menopause, 103, 128

Behavioral factors, 21, 45–47, 94–95, 105, 120. *See also* Abortion, induced; Birth control; Contraception; Sterilization

Beta distribution: for fecundability, 30, 33–34, 37; for intrauterine mortality, 73–74

Biometry, definition of, 2

Birth averted, 129

Birth control, 21, 105, 120, 121; bibliography of, 192–97; effect of, on fertility, 126, 128–30, 134. *See also* Abortion; Contraception; Sterilization

Birth intervals: by age at weaning (or at death), 89–90; bibliography of, 173; components of, 20, 85–92; by final size of family, 110–15, 148–57, 164–65; interior, 137–38; last, 37–38, 112–14, 149, 155, 166; open, 115, 138–39; straddling, 137–39; successive (closed), 110–15, 137–39, 149, 166; truncated, 89, 114

Breast-feeding, 21; bibliography of, 183–84; effect on fertility, 117–

20; effect on non-susceptible period, 82–91, 146; full vs. partial, 92–93, 134

Calendar rhythm method. *See* Ogino-Knaus method

Cellular division, 6–7, 78

Censored data, 33

Childlessness, 20

Chromosomal anomalies, 1, 45, 76–78

Cluster effect, 71, 103

Coefficient of variation: for birth intervals, 138; for fecundability, 36

Cohort, definition of, 51; life-table, 53

Coitus. *See* Sexual intercourse

Coitus interruptus, 126–27

Combinatorial analysis, 132

Competing events, 52

Completed fertility: birth intervals, 111–15; estimated through models, 115–19; number of births, 106–10, 147

Components of fertility: bibliography of, 176–77; definition of, 3, 16, 21